My
Mediterranean Village Lifestyle

RENA AYYELINA

TRAVELING BACK TO MY VILLAGE TO DISCOVER OPTIMAL HEALTH NATURALLY

WESTBOW
PRESS®
A DIVISION OF THOMAS NELSON
& ZONDERVAN

Scripture taken from the New King James Version®. Copyright ©
1982 by Thomas Nelson. Used by permission. All rights reserved.

WestBow Press books may be ordered through booksellers or by contacting:

WestBow Press
A Division of Thomas Nelson & Zondervan
1663 Liberty Drive
Bloomington, IN 47403
www.westbowpress.com
1 (866) 928-1240

ISBN: 978-1-5127-6820-6 (sc)

Print information available on the last page.

WestBow Press rev. date: 2/3/2017

CONTENTS

CHAPTER ONE

Discovering The Health Secrets of my Mediterranean Village

A man crosses a busy street and continues by foot several blocks to his favorite coffee shop, as has been his custom for the thirty-six years he has been retired; the man is 97 and takes no routine medicine. Who would not desire this degree of health at 97? How is it achieved? Is it a secret herb, a miracle pill, an ancient exercise secret or diet, or simply luck? Well, let's examine the man's life for clues.

My father rarely uses medicine and walked several blocks to his favorite καφενιο (coffee shop) even well into his nineties. Having grown up in a small village in Greece until the age of 52, my dad ate home cooked food that was fresh and seasonal. Eating seasonal food, as nature intended, provides maximum health benefits. Nearly everyone in the village had farmland to cultivate their crops including wheat. Most of what was eaten by the Lafkiotes (Λαυκιοτες, residents of Lafka, Λαυκα) was grown or raised in Lafka—out of necessity I might add.

Sheep and goats for milk, cheese, and occasional meat, and vegetables, fruit, wheat and olives were all produced locally. Rice and some pasta items that were easy to store and transport made their way to the village "general store." Other exceptions were coffee, sugar, and fish when the fishermen made an occasional trip to the village with their fresh catch to sell. Herbs such as oregano, parsley, bay leaf, and mint were used daily in cooking, as well as garlic, onion, cinnamon, nutmeg, and cloves; some were also used as medicine! Although nearly everyone had farmland, everyone gathered wild-growing items when they were available. Whatever was in season became the priority! I remember the women in the village would also gather wild dandelions for dinner. Picking dandelions remains common; we just witnessed the preparation of gathered dandelion greens on a recent trip back to Stymfalia (Στυμφαλια), which is a nearby village of some relatives. My father once took my husband and I up the mountain to pick oregano and tea. We walked up for about two hours and were well above the timberline when we arrived at the picking place. The aroma of both the tea and the oregano was quite robust. I also remember my family gathering snails after a good rain—you know, the escargot kind of snails! Financial necessity remained the main motivation for harvesting and gathering what was in season locally; however, as we will discuss further, it was a key component of the healthy Lafka village lifestyle.

Yianni (Γιαννη) lived in Greece his whole life, with the exception of nine years in America. Until age 52 he lived in Lafka, a mountain village. As I look back at my father's life, I can clearly see that circumstances changed in his life, but he did not change his diet that much. The most common work in Lafka was farming and raising sheep high in the mountains. Transportation was nearly all by foot, donkey or mule. Physical activity was a required part of daily living. No exercise class was necessary.

Because Greece is mostly rocky, the valuable flat land was used only for farming. The homes were built at the foot of the mountains. The traditional way to cultivate the land was with a plow and two mules. I still remember my parents walking to the fields at sun up to get as much done as possible before the midday heat. At around 11a.m. my parents would begin their walk back home to prepare and eat lunch, and they would take a nap until about 3p.m.

In addition to farming, everyone had small gardens at their house. Everyone grew food for his or her own family, and it was picked fresh and prepared in season without commercial processing. Because of this, it was packed with optimal nutrition! A significant portion of the village diet was fresh in-season items. What was coming in to season determined the menu. If you did not grow it, you probably would not have enough to survive. Unprocessed foods grown by someone else will give you the same benefits. Many families had a small vineyard and made their own wine. When I was growing up in Greece it was the norm for adults to have wine with dinner every night.

I was eleven when our family moved to the United States. The first few years of our restaurant business were very difficult financially. My parents worked tirelessly during this time, and my mother didn't have time to teach me what she knew about Greek home-cooked meals. Most of our time was spent making pizzas, which was our main business. As a result, I did not know how to cook when I got married. The first Greek dish I cooked, "pasticho," was horrible so we gave it to our dog Touko (an outside dog) to eat. My husband still makes fun of the fact that Touko barked at the dish that I slaved over to prepare! Lucky for me that after I had my children, an older Greek man that was a close friend of my parents, started visiting me. My parents had gone back to Greece by then, and he wanted to maintain friendships with Greek-speaking people—that would be me.

He often gave me advice on Greek cooking. The first cooking lesson was about oil. He said, "Greeks cook with extra virgin olive oil, not vegetable oils and lard! Of course, for citizens of Greece, cooking with olive oil is a no-brainer. Olives and olive oil have been a major industry of Greece and readily available for a very long time. Fortunate for the Greeks, and other Mediterranean countries, olive oil has been discovered to be the best, as recognized by almost all published experts. Among other qualities, it is rich in Omega-3 fatty acids and is a mono-unsaturated fat.

The water supply for the village came from deep inside the mountain. It was gathered in a reservoir and piped to all the homes. Unlike our chlorinated and fluoridated water, Lafka's water was clean and naturally full of minerals and absent of chemical runoff. I remember when I was a little girl, I used to go to the mountain to help with the sheep. There is also a fresh water spring there, called Kroeli (Κροελι), where I would bend over and drink water from. The water was ice cold even in the summer because it came directly from within the mountain. Our family vacations back to Lafka always included a family hike up the mountain to Kroeli. Even after a road was constructed instead of a path, we still walked instead of driving. Our kids loved packing a picnic lunch and dining beside the spring and enjoying the fresh, cold water.

My mother passed away at age 86 after suffering from diabetes, hypertension, a stroke, dementia, and finally heart failure. My mother began changing her diet when she came to America (age 47) and even more so after she retired (age 57). My parents then spent most of their time at their condominium in the city of Corinth, but my dad did not change his diet as much as my mother had while in the United States. When he retired and went back to Greece he ate the same as he had previously in Greece. He didn't raise crops, except for a small garden in Lafka, but he still ate fresh food in season. In Corinth you didn't go to a supermarket. You went in the center of town where a couple of blocks were lined up with produce stores, fish markets and meat markets. The produce was not refrigerated; it was fresh. The fish was brought in daily from the fisherman of Corinth. My parents were able to have fish more often while living in Corinth. The meat market had fresh, whole carcasses of sheep, goats, and chickens hanging.

Despite the easily available produce, my mother started eating a lot of sweets such as cake, ice cream, and candy. There are plenty of pastry and sweet shops (zaharoplastio in Greek) in Corinth. Almost every corner now has a zaharoplastio, and mother helped keep the shops in business. The sugary sweets were not an option when we lived in Lafka. Mother clearly became addicted to sugar, and she would do anything to get her poison. I remember one year I took my husband and children to Greece for a visit and saw my mom dip her finger in the honey and quickly put it in her mouth hoping no one saw her. She was so busy taking care of us that she did not have time to eat her sugar-rich snacks at her leisure, but she was going to get her sugar fix one way or another.

During most of their retirement, my parents would go back and forth between Corinth, where my mother preferred, and Lafka, where my father preferred. Lafka was the place to be during the hot Greek summers. It was much cooler and there was plenty of fresh, pure, cold water. Corinth was much more inviting during the colder months. It is warm enough to miss the Lafka snow and actually grow citrus, such as λεμονια (lemons) and πορτοκαλια (oranges). When leaving Corinth to stay in Lafka, they would load up with stuff from the markets in Corinth and take it to Lafka. As I said previous, if you lived in Lafka you pretty much ate what you or your neighbor grew. After retirement my father didn't farm; he rented his land out for a portion of the wheat. He did have a small garden for tomatoes, peppers, cucumbers etc. He maintained storage bins for his unprocessed wheat in his cellar. He also made his own Κρασι (wine) until his later years. When they went from Lafka to Corinth, they loaded down with Olive Oil, figs, wine, and cheese.

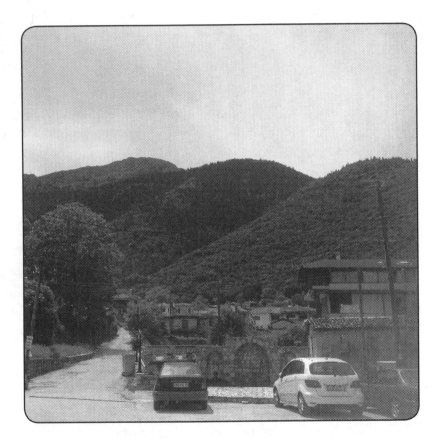

CHAPTER TWO

Quick and easy does not Work

Health: The World Health Organization (WHO) defined health in its broader sense in its 1948 constitution as, " A state of complete physical, mental, and social well-being and not merely the absence of disease or infirmity." Are you moving in the right direction? Are you moving towards a state of complete physical, mental, and social well-being? Are you moving toward longevity with a purposeful existence even in your 80's and 90's?

I am sure you have heard or read health comments like: eat fish for cancer protection, eating an avocado every day may help you reduce hunger, an apple a day keeps the doctor away, or eating a small serving of nuts every day reduces mortality by a certain percent. Although these foods help us to go the right direction towards better health, especially when these foods take the place of unhealthy choices, health is more complicated than eating a few of the right foods. There is no magic food, smoothie, or supplement that will improve our entire health and well-being or achieve that desired level of vitality. Doing one or two things towards a healthy lifestyle is like working the biceps daily to gain strength for the entire body. Exercising the biceps might make you gain strength in that muscle group, but it will not do much for the shoulders, back, abs, legs, core muscles, or any other part of the body.

I substitute teach at a group exercise facility, and I tell my group what muscles we are targeting for each particular exercise. I hear people saying, "I'm not eating healthy most days, but I am eating my protein bar full of vitamins and minerals and I am drinking plenty of water." Other people say to me, "I don't always eat healthy but I have a power shake every morning." If well-being and longevity only required doing one or two things, then staying healthy would be easy and simple. It is not a simple matter in today's society and economy; it's a lifestyle change. It's a difficult job taking control of your health, but the benefits are great and the cost of not doing it is of grave consequence. In the movie, *A Few Good Men,* I love the dialogue between Tom Cruise and Jack Nicholson: Nicholson: "I felt like his life might be in danger once word of the letter got out." Tom Cruise: "Grave danger?" Jack Nicholson; "Is there another kind?" If you take an honest look around at others, people you work around, family members, or friends, you surely see the grave consequences of poor health. They are grave consequences –grave as far as seriousness level and grave as far as destination.

Achieving health and longevity was not complicated for a "Lafkioti" (resident of Lafka). The lifestyle of necessity in Lafka (at that time) made health and longevity the natural outcome. In today's society and economy, if you live in an urban area or even a subdivision of sorts, healthy living is a little more complex; it requires action and a plan. It's about making an informed decision to journey towards living a life free of disease. That choice requires exerting the effort to understand healthy choices and avoiding the quick and easy way. That plan should include nutrition, exercise, avoiding toxins, spiritual life, and responsible medicine use when needed. If you become ill, take responsibility to investigate which type of treatment is best for you. Doris Day sang a hit song in the early sixties called, "Que sera sera (Whatever will be will be)." That may apply to many things, but that does not apply to achieving or maintaining your health. You must take control of your health because, otherwise, today's society and big-business will control your health. If you are reading this, you probably are not living in a village such as Lafka. You are probably not farming without a tractor, being physically active throughout the day, making your own cheese, and growing everything you eat.

We often tell our children not to take the easy way out because it does not pay in the long run; managing your health is the same concept. Which direction are you going? Here's a quote from Aristotle I love, "Good habits formed at youth make all the difference." We must choose God-created foods that are full of nutrition and free of toxins. The closer your food is to its origin, the better nutrition you will have, which means better health for you and your family. In Lafka, almost everyone in the village ate what they grew or raised. Even in this county before the industrial revolution people ate what they farmed and what livestock they raised on their farms. I know that a lot of us cannot go buy farms and recreate that lifestyle, but we can make necessary changes to go the right direction. Companies and the government are not, and should not be, accountable for our health and our family's health. We are accountable, and the earlier we accept this responsibility the faster we can move in the right direction and improve our health and our loved one's health.

Here are some quick-start suggestions to get started towards the right direction:

- First week: Start eating a healthy breakfast if you eat breakfast. If not, eat a healthy snack between 9-10 am.
- Second week: Add fresh or frozen fruit daily and change it up so by the end of the two weeks you have tried five or six different types of fruit.

- Third week: Eat at least one fresh or frozen vegetable daily prepared with extra virgin olive oil and change it up so by the end of the two weeks you have tried five or six different types of vegetables.
- Fourth week: Add sweet potatoes in your diet two or three times a week-- baked, broiled, or fried in extra virgin olive oil.
- Fifth week: Drink filtered (not plastic bottles) water -one glass 30 minutes or more before breakfast with fresh lemon juice. Drink another glass of water at mid-morning. Drink another glass of water before lunch. Drink another glass of water mid-afternoon. Drink another glass of water during dinner preparation. Drink another glass of water 30 minutes after dinner.
- Sixth week: Cook at home with God created ingredients at least 5 days a week, and make enough for lunch the next day. For example, if you make baked sweet potatoes, throw an extra in for lunch the next day and add some vegetables and you are good to go. Also very important, cook before you get hungry, as my mom use to say.
- Seventh week: Eat a handful of raw nuts for one of your snacks daily.
- Leave the table almost full especially if you eat fast. If you are still hungry in 30 minutes eat a little more.

You are on your way to "a state of complete physical, mental, and social well-being and not merely the absence of disease or infirmity." Keep making improvements to your diet, and as the improvements become habits, you will start feeling better and feeling better about yourself. Once you are at that triumphant milestone, you will be motivated to learn even more ways to enhance the healthier you!

CHAPTER THREE

Common Myths About a Healthy Lifestyle

- **"Health declines over age fifty"**

A healthy human lifespan should be about one hundred years. It's sad, but true, that poor health at fifty or older is often a result of lifestyle choices. We reduce ourselves to "sick care" instead of taking control of our health. Yes we have advanced in drugs, surgical procedures, and medical technology, and that is to our benefit; however, what about our lifestyle? Does our diet consist of processed foods that alter nutritional value with harmful chemicals and preservatives? Are we living an active lifestyle or a sedentary lifestyle? What about our environment? Is the air that we breathe in our homes polluted with cleaning chemicals, paint, mold, pet dander, or chemical air fresheners. What about our stress level? Are we managing our stress levels or merely reacting to our stress levels? With modest and progressive adjustments to lifestyle, health and longevity can be more than just a dream. I challenge each of you to invest in your health (and your family's) starting today. If you already have a healthy lifestyle, I challenge you to continually reassess your daily choices in light of what you are learning and keep moving forward.

- **"My family has to participate"**

It would be great if we could get our family members to change their behavior to better health choices at the same time we did, but most of the time this is not realistic. People don't change habits because we demand that they change; they often want to see the change in someone else, like us. This is the case with almost any habit change, and healthy lifestyle choices are no exception. You have to start the lifestyle changes and lead by example; example is what most effectively influences others. They may not participate 100% initially, but by watching the positive effects that behavior change and purposeful decisions are having on your life, it's more likely that your family will follow. I love this well-known saying, "Don't talk, just act. Don't say, just show. Don't promise, just prove." Get started today and believe that something amazing is about to happen when you make the decision to eat healthy, exercise, and spend time in prayer. Believe that you will feel better, your skin will look younger, you will have more energy, and you will wake up with a positive attitude towards life. How to get started? Have faith that you will overcome the bad lifestyle habits. You will start making those necessary healthy lifestyle changes based on your dialogue with yourself. When your family starts seeing the positive effects your changes have made, they will find it hard not to at least give it their best effort. No more excuses; just do it!

- **"I'm too young or too old to start a healthy lifestyle"**

Disease can strike at any age. It's scary, but unfortunately true, that some diseases hit the very young. Some examples are cancer and type II diabetes that can hit even in childhood. Parents have the responsibility to teach their kids the importance of nutrition, exercise, prayer, and abstaining from destructive habits such as smoking and recreational drugs. Remember, kids watch their parents, so what you say to your children you must practice. The elderly can improve their health through diet and exercise also. Many elderly people feel that it is too late for them to improve their health, but that is simply not true. Let's look at a couple of examples of disease that are common late in life. Osteoporosis is one of those diseases, and you can minimize or avoid its destruction by regular exercise and getting out in the sun for 15-30 minutes in the morning before 10 a.m. or in the afternoon after 4 p.m. Arthritis is another disease that can be minimized with regular exercise, getting to a healthier weight, and eating foods that are rich in omega-3 fatty acids. It's never too late to make healthier lifestyle changes so you can enjoy life.

I watched a report about the transformation of an elderly bear that was rescued from roadside circus (Yahoo News, March 9, 2016). The transformation was "astonishing" per the report. The before pictures showed how skinny the bear was, and her fur was white, thin and dirty. She also suffered from painful untreated arthritis. After being rescued and taken care of, it only took months for her body to change to a healthy bear, and her legs to start getting stronger every day. Her fur regained its normal color and density. She, for the first time in her life, at the age of 30, was allowed to hibernate. The bear is now living a very happy, and healthy life (as a senior) in her new protected natural environment. What were some of the specific factors that had brought the bear her crippling condition and near death? The bear was kept in a small cage with a concrete floor. That means no exercise or autonomy of action, and resulting depression. The bear couldn't hibernate because of the environment and restrictions on activity. That means the bear was totally stressed and tired. People get that way if they don't get enough sleep. In captivity the bear was not allowed to eat its normal diet, which is the healthiest diet for a bear. We can learn about lifestyle changes even from wild animals. Education is a key to a healthier you, so be a lifetime learner.

- **"Healthy food is tasteless, boring food"**

In my community, one or more of five ingredients-- fat, salt, sugar, cheese, or barbecue sauce, seasons the majority of food. Many people cannot name more than a handful of spices. You can read more about some of the common spices used in Lafka in chapter eleven. In chapter eleven you will read about the health benefits of some of those spices. So going back to the common seasoning used here in the Ohio Valley region, you should know that they are all items that you shouldn't have too much of. Much of the fat around here is from deep-frying, which is commonly accepted as being bad for your health. Sugar and excessive salt are not good either; both are discussed further later. Real cheese without added ingredients can be part of a healthy diet and supplies protein and calcium; however, it is not healthy to melt it all over everything you eat. Barbecue sauce is not inherently bad for you if made with good ingredients and spices, but that is not what most people use. Some things are an acquired taste. My husband used to savor all of that melted cheese, but he has now acquired a taste for herbs and spices and does not use cheese on everything now. Healthy food does not have to be boring!

- **"Egg yolk has high cholesterol, and it's bad for your health"**

My mother would pack hard-boiled eggs for my lunch when I went to school in Greece, and she would pack us hard-boiled eggs when my brother and I went to the mountain in the summer to tend to our sheep. We had chickens, so fresh eggs were available and because hard-boiled eggs stay good for days, it was an great option along with feta cheese, olives, and home-made bread for a packed lunch. I always told my mom that I wanted mine with the yolk soft because I loved dipping my bread in the yolk; it was delicious. We ate meat only about once a week, so eggs provided the added protein we needed. What happened to the egg yolk? For most of my adult life in America I have heard bad things about cholesterol. There have been those saying you should only eat a small number of eggs per week as a result of "cholesterol fear." A lot of people stopped eating egg yolks, including two people in my family because of the reports that came out "research shows...." I did not stop eating egg yolk because it did not make common sense to eat only egg white! Seriously, I could not understand why my family members, along with a lot of other people would buy these cartons with egg white. The thought of buying eggs in a carton without any of the nutrition of the yolk seemed wrong to me.

Recently we began hearing that research shows that eggs (the whole egg) are good for your health in moderation. Eggs provide many important nutrients: vitamins A, D, E, K, B6, B12, thiamine and minerals calcium, iron, phosphorus, and zinc. Eggs also provide essential fatty acids. My suggestion is to eat an egg every day if you want unless you are following a specific diet prescribed to you by your health provider. I generally eat one per day or two every other day. Currently many are beginning to realize that the cholesterol in eggs is not as much of a concern as cholesterol associated the saturated fats from animal fats. With what we understand now about some types of saturated fats, overly processed foods, trans-fats and hydrogenated oils, I believe it is more important to avoid excesses of sausage, bacon, and hash browns (unless made from fresh potatoes and cooked in good oil) and to avoid margarine completely!

A multitude of Americans are on "statins," which are cholesterol-lowering drugs. My husband recently shared a conversation he had with a physician friend who had "borderline high" total cholesterol, as is my husband's level (note-my husbands good cholesterol AKA HDL is way high-82). My husband's doctor friend said that, "Most doctors think everybody needs to be on a statin." He added that, "It's out of control!" He had been talked into trying statins but quit taking them because they made him "not feel good." The doctor friend acknowledged that some people should be on them, but that it is not reasonable that so many people are on them. Massive advertising has convinced a whole generation that the pill is the answer. Don't quit taking medication without discussing with your physician, but educate yourself so it is actually a discussion. Despite your decision after your conversation with your physician and your research, everyone can benefit from good nutrition and lifestyle choices and habits.

CHAPTER FOUR

Healthy Children

Every aspect of your child's health begins at home; that includes nutritional habits. If children see their parents making good decisions, they are much more likely to make good decisions later in life. Children learn to eat healthy by participating in family meals that are healthy. Eating junk food and expecting your child to make healthy choices is about the same as smoking and having a surprised look when your child starts smoking.

My departed friend from the island of Kalymnos, used to say to me, "The first lesson for your children is at home, not at school." He did not have a degree from high school, but he apparently had a degree in life's lessons. Life's lessons can be from successes or failures. Some of the most significant life lessons come from failures. There is a saying I have heard often, but I don't know its origin that says, "A foolish person does not learn from his mistakes, a smart person learns from his mistakes, but a wise person learns from the mistakes of others." Look around at the life and health of others around you and in society. Do you think about their health issues and learn from their lifestyles about choices to avoid, or will you wait until a personal health crisis to learn? My friend from Kalymnos lived alone and a lot of the time he looked like a homeless man because he did not have the best clothes or a nice car, but he had common sense and a lot of wisdom that he freely shared to anyone that would listen to him (and some that wouldn't listen to him). My friend didn't necessarily make all of the best choices in life, but was willing to share lessons he had learned. Many of his shared lessons were about raising children. It's important to start the kids on healthy food from day one because it's very hard to change their dietary habits later in life, and even harder for them to obtain or maintain good health as adults.

When my children's friends would come to our house to visit and play with my kids, I would always include some fruit with whatever snack I prepared for them. I will never forget some of the comments some of the kids would make about the fruit— "like, what is it? Do I peel it? Is it good?" And believe me, some of them would spit it out because they were not used to the taste. Unfortunately, a lot of kids have never tasted fruits like apricots, kiwi, cherries, and pomegranates to name a few.

My girlfriend, originally from Cyprus, still remembers coming to my house with her kids when I got off work so the kids could play together. I would not allow my kids to eat snacks until they ate their prepared foods including their vegetables. Thank God I was given the wisdom from my old friend from Kalymnos to rediscover the village diet I experienced as a young child. That experience compelled me to feed the kids healthy food, and now that they are adults you will not see junk food in their house. My husband and I worked full time and then some while we were raising our children, but we always made raising our children a priority, and this definitely included nutrition and cooking as a priority.

My husband didn't really cook, but he would give the baths and help ensure homework was done so I could focus on dinner. It was during this time that my husband began his continuing habit of preparing breakfast. During the early years I went to work earlier than my husband. He would prepare the kids breakfast and take them to school. Although we didn't do everything right and continue to learn about nutrition, he did cook eggs and breakfast sandwiches often and avoided all of the sugar of popular cereals. I would also pack their lunch if they were going to the babysitter to ensure my kids did not eat processed meats, chips and cookies. It was hard work because even people in our family would make fun of me and feed them junk food when I was not around. In the 80's, and 90's you did not hear a lot about health in general, but I had roots from Lafka that taught me what healthy food looks like. Children's health is a concern in America now because of poor choices in lifestyle and nutrition, much of it caused by marketing by huge corporations.

Childhood obesity is on the rise, and so is childhood disease. We have neglected to teach them to eat healthy because we, the adults, have unhealthy lifestyles ourselves. Are you content to continue floating down stream with the driftwood and dead fish, or are you willing to swim upstream to gain better health for you and your family? Is it not alarming to hear that children are getting some of the diseases that adults usually have such as: cancer, type 2 diabetes, and high blood pressure? Why should a child have high blood pressure—really? It should scare us to death! It should wake us up to take inventory of our kitchen cabinets, our pantries, our refrigerators, and our freezers and to question our convenient stops at the fast food restaurant. Do you ever wonder what does it take to alarm us?

Grandparents can be a significant influence on a child's life. Don't take the easy way out by buying cheap, addictive food and snacks for your grandchildren; you put their health at risk and increase their chances of starting a chronic health condition early in life. Take responsibility and help the parents promote healthy food choices instead of having the common mentality, " When at grandparents house you are spoiled, and sent back to your parents at the end of the day for them to deal with it." This is simply wrong thinking; grandparents share in the responsibility to raise healthy children free from disease. Don't feed a child junk and ask God why they are stricken with disease later.

Parents and grandparents have a meaningful and lasting influence on a child's health! Below are some suggestions to raise healthy children:

- Allow the children to help with meals, not just to help with the clean up. It's fun for them to help cook a meal and perhaps they will have a better attitude when asked to help with the clean up.
- Take the children to the supermarket to help with the selection of healthy foods and explain why you choose one type of food over another.
- Take the children to a farm to see how crops and livestock are raised.
- If possible, grow a garden together, even if it is a small "container" garden.
- Children need also exercise for their health, so take them to the parks, ride a bike together, play ball in the back yard, walk in the neighborhood, go fishing together...

There are many fun activities to do with children to keep them active and to make beautiful memories together. Have you ever heard anyone say that they wish they had spent more time watching television or playing video games? Have you ever heard a middle-aged person say they were so glad they started smoking as a child or teenager? Do you think you will look back and say, "I wish I would have had less home-cooked dinners at home with my family and had went to the drive through more often?" The three questions are really the same; your diet and lifestyle can rob your child's health just as smoking will rob your child's health.

CHAPTER FIVE

Your Health is Your Wealth!

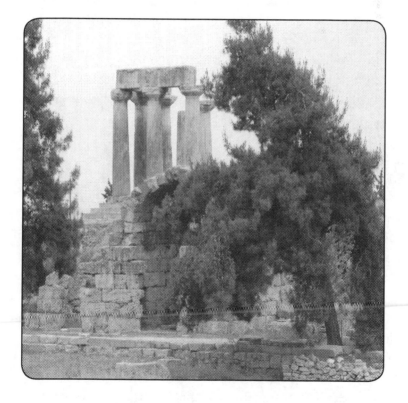

Am I going to have enough money for retirement? We worry a lot about wealth accumulation and retirement planning, but what about "real wealth management?" Real wealth is your health! Will you have enough health-wealth to do what you want during retirement? You can travel the world over for the cost of one hospitalization and have pocket money afterwards! Think about it.

So let's talk about what you want to do in retirement. I bet you want to be the best Bunko player in the nursing home—right? But that's later; first when you retire in your sixties you want to travel somewhere nice and see it from the bus with a bunch of other people who also can't walk because they have arthritis, high blood pressure, heart conditions, or are just overweight, underactive and hoping the tour includes a donut shop or a buffet. If that is you, you have bought the wrong book. If that is not you, you probably want to do things a bit differently. You probably want to still be agile and active and do healthy activities with your grandchildren. Maybe you want to see the world and realize the world is a little farther away from the bus tour or the boat tour. Maybe you want to do more of hobbies you couldn't when you were working. Skiing, cross-country biking, hiking or maybe even mountain biking might be what stokes your fire.

Traveling the world off of the beaten tourist path is my dream. My husband and I had such a great time backpacking in France. I don't mean backpacking in the woods. I mean backpacking from city to city by foot and train. I didn't even realize what I was missing until my husband took us there for our anniversary. My husband had first taken a couple of backpacking trips to Europe with our adult son. That got started because my son was going to venture there by himself, which we didn't think was safe. My son was glad to have his dad along. The point to this is this; if my husband had not been in good physical shape and able to walk with a full pack for miles each day, he would not have had the chance. That means our trips together traveling would not have been possible either. Do you have enough health-wealth to seize the day when it comes around? I didn't mention my husband's other passion he wants to continue pursuing in retirement. It is mountain biking!

I am talking black diamond and double-black diamond trails in his upper fifties and beyond. I am not telling you to mountain bike. You might break a rib like my husband, but he healed up and got back in the saddle.

Ok, enough about what we like to do. The point, again, is this. A healthy enjoyable retirement is more than just quitting work and taking it easy. If you don't use it, you will lose it. In fact, you will lose it quickly. Staying active is just part of the investment you must make to show a good return on your investment for retirement. Good nutritional and lifestyle choices are the other components necessary for an awesome retirement.

Investing in your health is a wise decision, and one that leads to optimal health for a long time. Let us again consider Yianni, my dad. He only takes medicine on rare occasions and that didn't start until well into his nineties. The question is, what are you waiting for? Is it your next symptom, your next doctor's appointment, your next x-ray, or your next colonoscopy? You are 100% accountable for healthy eating decisions. When you take the responsibility and stop blaming your genes, your spouse, the food corporations, the restaurants…. you will begin to choose quality food that nourishes your body. I'm often surprised when people say, "I can't afford healthy food because it's expensive." Many of these same people choose to drive new and/or expensive cars, have the latest cell phone or computer, carry designer purses, and go out to dinner several nights a week, but they prefer to buy cheap groceries.

The decision is yours; just ask yourself the question, "Do I want a healthier (aka wealthier) life for myself and my family?" I thank God we live in a country where we can still make most free choices. The free choice to live healthy is yours, and yours alone. If the answer is yes, you must take an active role; you must accept accountability. Being healthy is not a one-day on, one-day off decision, it's a healthy lifestyle everyday. If your family is not willing to make those healthier choices, be the "example" and they will notice the positive changes such as: better mood, increased energy, a positive attitude, reduction in weight, and a good night's sleep.

Your health is a serious endeavor and there is no time to waste; however, transforming your lifestyle into a healthy one will not happen overnight, especially if you have a family. Pay attention and get this crucial point! Your commitment to change must be made overnight; do not put it off. You can't become a marathon runner overnight, but there is a point at which you must make a commitment. Like a marathon runner, you may become tired and want to quit along the way and pull up beside the drive through window instead of walking through the grocery produce section, but you must press on to be a winner. If you improve your health and your family's health, you are the champion! Don't choose to continue to be the loser.

So let's start this marathon in the kitchen with some healthy, basic ingredients, but first, take out the trash. Trash everything that has ingredients that you cannot pronounce. Now you have room for the good stuff!

Must have ingredients for the healthy conscience cook:

- Extra virgin olive oil in a 3L can—you need a larger container because healthy cooking is more than sprinkling some on your salad, although that is good.
- Real butter—step away from the margarine. If you don't believe me, look at the ingredients and do your own research.

- Cinnamon – nothing better than the smell of cinnamon when added to a recipe, especially the type you bake. Cinnamon is also a healthy spice. I prefer Ceylon cinnamon because it's superior to the cheaper cassia. See chapter eleven for more about cinnamon.
- Whole-wheat pasta and spaghetti - Delicious and with lots of fiber! What a great way to keep things moving in your digestive system, and help protect you from cancer.
- Whole-wheat non-GMO (genetically modified) flour - most of us have the need to use flour in our recipes; why not make it a nutritious food item? Throw out that unhealthy white flour and let's get healthy.
- Honey - Throw out that margarine/easy spread... and lightly spread some delicious and nutritious honey on that toast and sprinkle some cinnamon on it too! Did you know that honey was called "Nectar of the gods" in Greek mythology?
- Oregano - most Greeks including me can't cook without it. Along with the many health benefits, oregano is a flavorful addition to salads, soups, roast and more. A Greek village tomato salad with dried oregano, feta cheese, cucumbers, and extra virgin olive oil is one of my favorite salads that my mom used to make. She would crush the dried oregano leaves between her fingers and the sweet aroma was released in the air. See chapter eleven for more about oregano.
- Inexpensive red and white wine to use in your recipes.
- Parsley
- Vinegar - there is a lot of information out there to drink it by the spoonful and its benefits. Personally I use my village's common sense on vinegar. Vinegar is delicious when used to enhance flavor in your dishes, and because you will love the taste this way as opposed to the spoonful

method, you will use it often. A Healthy food also has to taste good or most people will not add it to their diet.

- Fresh lemons —please squeeze the real lemon instead of buying a plastic lemon container with juice in it.

My mother-in-law made a wise comment one day as we were leaving a medical complex, "This parking lot is full! A lot of people must be sick." Even though my beautiful mother-in-law that I love and admire very much was diagnosed with Alzheimer's and has little short-term memory, she is wise enough to notice a medical complex parking lot full of people is an indicator that too many people are sick. We really need to wake up and notice when the medical complex parking lots are consistently more full than the farmer's market, organic grocers, or children's playgrounds and parks. Can you see that it is time to start making much needed changes to your family's lifestyle?

CHAPTER SIX

Dine Out Without Pigging-Out

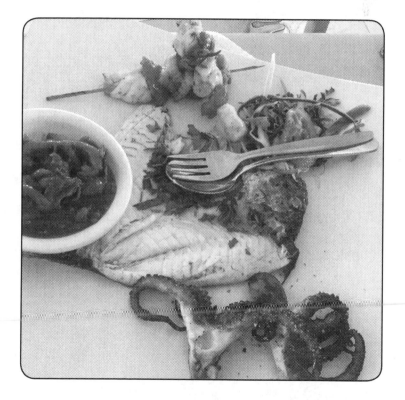

Dining out occasionally and staying healthy can be done. The well-known adage, "Knowledge is power," is true in regards to health also. I have seen a lot of people order a dish smothered with cheese and order a diet cola to go with that meal. Each time you order at a restaurant, each time you reach into your cabinet, each time you reach into your refrigerator, you basically decide whether you will build a strong immune system or you will weaken your immune system. I love to read Greek philosophy. One day I came upon this quote that I live by, "The part can never be well unless the whole is well." -Plato

Don't think of dining at a restaurant as a chance to "punish the buffet" or "pig out!" You were created to graze, not gorge. It's not necessary to have a menu with the calories listed to make wise, healthy choices, and taste does not have to be compromised either.

Here are some suggestions when dining out:

- Don't order appetizers; if you are still hungry you can order an appetizer later. Most people eat the appetizers and are half full when the entrée arrives. Then you feel that you need to eat it all since you have paid for it.
- Ask the server to bring the breadbasket at the same time the food comes.
- Choose baked, broiled or grilled entrees instead of deep-fried dishes.
- Ask the server to bring the dressing for the salad on the side so you can decide how much to use.
- Ask the server to bring the butter for that potato on the side so you can decide how much to use.
- Don't starve all day when you have plans to go out to eat; this will tempt you to gorge.
- Dining out does not mean you have to eat until you are so stuffed that walking to the car is a difficult task and each subsequent breath reminds you that you ate too much again.

- When the server asks, "Do you want a cookie for just $1 more?", say, "No thanks." You will feel better, and most importantly, you will stay healthy.
- When the server says, "Would you like to up-size that order?", say, "No thanks." Remember that you are grazing, not gorging. If you are hungry later, you don't have to go chase down a deer for something to eat. This is civilization; you have a refrigerator! If you lived in a society where you did have to go chase down a deer to eat, then gorging might work for you, but not here. Not in today's society. Respect your body because it's the only one you will ever have here on earth.

You are paying good money for a dining experience, and you should enjoy the experience and feel good about it. Since you are what you eat, you should leave the restaurant feeling good about whom you are.

CHAPTER SEVEN

The Labels of Processed Foods Should Have to List Side Effects

Take control of your health. In my group exercise classes the instructor asks the class if anyone has a need that we can all pray for before we start exercising. I am saddened and shocked as to how many people ask for prayer for someone with cancer. Per the American Cancer Society, "Cancer remains the second most common cause of death in the US, accounting for nearly 1 of every 4 deaths." The American Cancer Society also recognizes the importance of good nutrition, exercise and lifestyle choices in preventing cancer and provides information for each. I believe the father of medicine when he said, "All disease begins in the gut." – Hippocrates. We don't have a cure for cancer. Diabetes, heart disease, and suicide due to depression to name a few are also on the rise in the United States. There are thousands of chemicals approved by the FDA to be used in our so-called food, and many new ones added each year. We need a label on the processed food listing the side effects. If people would cut out processed foods we would see a big decrease in disease. You have been taught that annual exam is part of health care. My good friend told me yesterday that she is going for her annual exam next week. I had to ask the question, why? She said because she wants to ensure everything is okay with her health. My friend eats the Greek diet, she spends time with family, friends, and goes to church to nourish her soul, but she does not exercise, which is a very important part of maintaining health. What are you doing between annual exams to maintain or restore health? Ask yourself these questions:

- Am I providing my body with the nutrients it needs to build healthy cells? Your diet should consist of mostly unprocessed food (shoot for 80%), and most of it in fruits and vegetables.
- Am I exercising at least 3 times a week and doing what I can to keep moving the other days. Sitting for long periods is not healthy even if you exercise strenuously at times.
- Am I feeding my soul? The craving deep in your soul is a craving for God's Word. It is a call to read the Holy Scriptures. As Jesus said, "Man shall not live by bread alone, but by every word that proceeds from the mouth of God" (Matthew 4:4, NKJV).

A lot of people ask me if I take supplements. The answer is yes! Why? Because due to modern farming methods, even the best diet lacks some of the vitamins and minerals your body needs. Additionally, nutritional need is up due to our toxic environment and the excess stress of our society. This chapter isn't about stress, but it must be managed if you have a stressful lifestyle or profession. I remember when my parents used sheep manure to fertilize their fields and olive trees. Modern farming methods use synthetic fertilizers, along with pesticides, herbicides, and insecticides. These methods can strip the soil of nutrients, and put humans at higher risk of health problems such as cancer. If we want to decrease disease and increase optimal health, we must return to the way God intended for us to cultivate the soil. God's plan called for letting the soil rest (Leviticus 25:4) every seventh year. Nothing rests these days it seems. We think crop rotation, fertilizer, herbicides and pesticides take care of it all.

CHAPTER EIGHT

Gift Wrapping Wonderland

It's fun to receive and to give gifts wrapped in pretty paper and a beautiful ribbon. The thrill of seeing a beautiful package with our name on it, and wondering what it could be, is exciting. When we finally open the present, we may or may not be thrilled about what it actually is. You have probably had occasions when the gift was beautifully packaged, but what it contained wasn't what you really wanted or needed. Yes, you appreciated the thought behind it, but you just didn't know how you would use it.

We can also apply the gift-wrapping wonderland to packaged foods and processed foods. Have you noticed how companies entice us by the beautiful package? It's not an accident; packaging design has the primary goal of grabbing your attention, and some companies spend millions on logo and package design. It's often the packaging and display that sells the product more than what is actually in it. Once we open the package, does it taste as good as the marketing said it would? More importantly, does our body know how to use it as fuel and for cellular repair? The food we eat is the substance our body uses for our essential physical and mental functions.

A surprise gift for your birthday, anniversary, or Christmas is an exciting and good thing generally; however, surprise ingredients in food is almost never a good thing. More stuff for your birthday is good, but more stuff in your food is always bad. Look at the ingredients listed on the label of the five most common processed foods you eat. Ask yourself the purpose of the chemicals and otherwise modified "food substances." And there is more to worry about than the added ingredients listed. Some potentially harmful chemicals, below some arbitrary limit that a bureaucracy set, do not even have to be listed. These "less than significant" threshold levels often utilized research conducted by the large company that stands to benefits from using it.

There is a connection between food and disease. In order to prevent disease we must not look at the pretty package; we must look at the ingredients that make up that food item if we want to give our bodies the proper fuel to function at an optimal level. If your goal is to become healthy, you must take charge of your own destiny! You must return to eating foods that your great-grandmother prepared and ate--no more just grabbing convenient pretty packaging full of ingredients that actually rob from our health account. Make deposits in your health account by choosing more and more unprocessed foods. To the extent that you must consume processed foods, read all the ingredients? If your great-grandmother would not recognize the ingredients as food, then it's probably not the present your body wants; it is likely just pretty packaging and marketing. They are probably ingredients that increase the profit margin without consideration for your health. But in all fairness to the companies, it is really not their responsibility to improve your health. It is your responsibility; do not delegate this responsibility. Here are some easy steps you can use for healthier grocery shopping:

- Stay in the perimeter of the grocery store first, then to the frozen section (select items with only one ingredient) and then go to the remaining isles if you must. The fresh, healthy foods unadulterated by processing and additives are found in the perimeter, and by the time you get finished there, you should have selected most of your groceries (and nutrients).

- Read all ingredients
- Look below eye-level of the grocery shelves because in that area is where the expensive and leading brands are found and not necessarily the healthy items.
- Leave the children at home, or plan to educate them in nutrition as you take them to the grocery store. Corporations spend millions developing packaging that appeals to the kids. Don't let corporations determine your child's level of health; that is your job! Step up to the plate!
- Dress nice before going grocery shopping, because it's fun and will boost your mood! What we wear doesn't give us health, but let's be honest for a moment. Don't you want to look healthy, be healthy, and display vitality and a robust enthusiasm for life?

It's time for me to do my grocery shopping now if my hard working husband is going to eat this evening. He always looks forward to my Mediterranean cooking with a splash of American and Chinese stir-fry. "Ta leme." (talk soon in Greek)

CHAPTER NINE

Misleading Food Labels

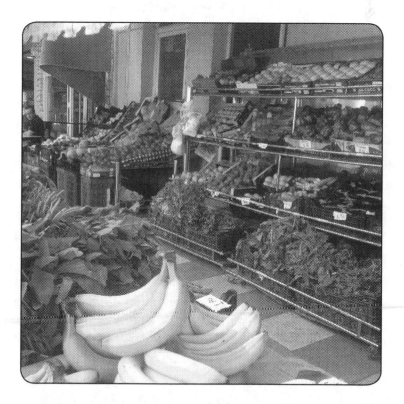

Eat the foods you love, but with real ingredients!

Most people don't realize that their food choices create their
health problems. In fact, your food choices can be unknowingly
robbing you of your health-wealth even if you don't yet have a

clue you have lost some health or potential for continuing health. Just because a label on the front claims to be healthy, low fat, fat free, nutritious, natural…does not mean it's a good food product. The claims can be misleading phrases used by the company to grab your attention. Often the added ingredient that reduces fat is more sugar, which is bad. The added ingredient to reduce sugar is artificial sweetener, which is bad. You can't just focus on "low fat" or "low sugar." You shouldn't eat a lot of some types of fat, and you certainly shouldn't eat a lot of sugar. But you are much better off developing some self-control and eating real ingredients in moderation than trusting your health to a chemical company. By the time that someone figures out (because a lot of people have developed cancer etc.) that a chemical additive is bad for you, it is too late. Eat the real stuff, knowing that too much of some things is not good, and at least know and see the results instead of waiting for a chronic or terminal illness to develop. A lot of people usually have to suffer before the dots can be connected to form a picture showing it is harmful. And then, some companies will hide or fight the results as long as they can.

I have heard several discussions that pointed out the truth that curing disease is not profitable, and I agree. The money is in treating chronic disease. Look at the television pharmaceutical adds. Do you see any for life saving antibiotics for the "superbugs" threatening us? No you don't, and here is why. The pharmaceutical companies want a big return on their research investment for their stockholders, so they focus on drugs for chronic health conditions, not ones you get cured of and move on to health. You know, the stuff that you must continue taking drugs for to be "healthy." Don't worry about eating huge chili-dogs, just keep taking the medicine for heartburn. Don't eat healthy and make lifestyle changes to reduce your cholesterol level, just take statin drugs. Clearly there is something wrong, because we are eating foods with no fat, low fat, low salt, no salt, and still have a serious problem with obesity in this country. Let's examine some misleading labels.

- **Whole Grains and Real fruit filling** - The ingredients are too many to list, but here's the first few: High-fructose corn syrup, corn syrup, strawberry puree concentrate, sugar, glycerin, maltodextrin, sodium alginate, modified cornstarch, methylcelluloce, citric acid, monocalcium phosphate, xanthan gum, malic acid, red 40...and the list goes on.
- **Fruit flavored snacks** - Ingredients: Corn syrup, sugar, apple puree concentrate, water, modified corn starch, gelatin, contains 2% or less of citric acid, vitamin C (ascorbic acid), artificial flavor, red 40.
- **Butter flavored syrup** - Some of the ingredients are: Corn syrup, high fructose corn syrup, water, contains less than 2% of salt, cellulose gum, natural and artificial flavors, sodium hexamataphosphate, sodium benzoate, and sorbic acid (preservatives), caramel color.
- **Fat free** - fat free yogurt has 17 grams of sugar. Regular yogurt has only 9 grams of sugar.
- **Almond milk, 90 calories vs. Organic whole milk** - Almond milk has 16 grams of sugar/Organic whole milk has 11 grams of sugar.
- **Whole wheat bread** - Some of the ingredients are: sugar, vital wheat gluten, molasses, lecithin, sodium stearoyl lactylate, calcium propionate, datem, monocalcium phosphate, ammonium sulfate.
- **"Healthy" spreads** - Some of the ingredients are: oil blends, whey, artificial flavors, lecithin, emulsifiers, and preservatives.
- **Avocado oil barbeque potato chips** - Some of the ingredients are: Avocado oil, sugar, salt, dextrose, tomato powder, dried honey, (honey, evaporated cane juice),

brown sugar, spices, yeast extract, onion powder, natural flavors, extractives of paprika, caramel color, citric acid. Note: some ingredients like caramel color are not as innocent as they sound. Let's take Caramel color possible ingredients: "Caramel coloring can be made from a variety of carbohydrates including: dextrose (corn), invert sugar, malt syrup (barley), molasses, lactose (sugar in milk), starch hydrolysates (corn or wheat). What is invert sugar? Invert sugar is a sugar mixture that has been chemically altered to make it sweeter than table sugar.

- **Lunch ready packages for kids -** Some of the ingredients are (too many to list them all on this one particular package so I will list the ingredients my grandmother would not recognize as food): glycerin, soybean oil, wheat gluten, mono-& diglycerides, artificial flavor, potassium sorbate, xanthan gum, cellulose powder, sodium citrate, corn syrup, maltodextrin, dextrose, partially hydrogenated soybean oil, red 40, blue 1, yellow 3, yellow 5.

- **A multi grain cereal -** Some of the ingredients are: Sugar, corn syrup, trisodium phosphate, malic acid.

CHAPTER TEN

Redefining Home Cooked Meals

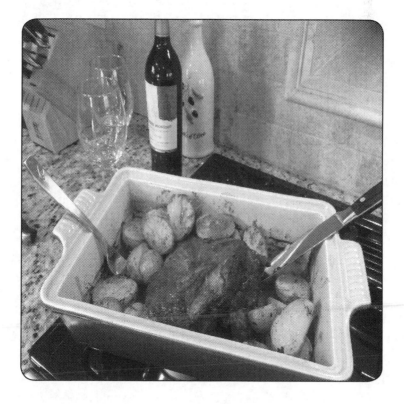

You have seen the recipes called "quick and easy meals." The meals are not described as "healthy" (and should not be), just quick and easy. What keeps the meals and recipes from being healthy? Most recipes call for opening of cans and bags of processed foods and adding a couple of fresh ingredients before mixing it up and baking. This is not a home cooked meal. This is processed food added together and baked.

My parents used to visit us once a year after they first retired and went back to Greece. Mother would watch me cook for the family and was stunned at what I called a home cooked meal. I remember her exact comment to my dad one day, she said, "Yianni, look what your daughter is calling a home cooked meal! She is opening cans, warming the contents and serving us a home cooked meal." My mother did not have time to teach me how to cook when I was a teenager, and if she did I would not have listened anyway. I learned to cook from my mother-in-law, my friends, and a cookbook written in the 1970's. My mother-in-law took every processed food shortcut she learned about. Advertisements for soups pointed to recipes for casseroles based on canned soup. Friends offered their secret recipes using processed food shortcuts. Marketing from large food companies made the pitch to a whole generation of women. This is how they could save time and still be the "cook" of the family. This is what almost an entire generation was programmed to do, and also to eat!

Greek cooking, as I left it when I immigrated to the U.S., consists mainly of fresh ingredients. The dishes changed with seasonal bounty in my village of Lafka. Whatever was in season was what we ate. It was packed with nutrition because it was fresh; we never ate processed food. The solution to our health crisis in America is to go back and eat like the Greeks did 40-50 years ago. So how can we adopt this diet? Let's get started with some actionable tips to help at the grocery:

- First, do eighty percent of your shopping around the perimeter of the grocery store where the fresh foods and the one-ingredient frozen foods generally are. If you are like me, you are on a budget. Since you spent the majority of your budget on fresh or frozen foods, it will eliminate the temptation to buy too many processed foods.

- Maximize the nutrition value by choosing a variety of colors in fruit and vegetables.
- Read all of the ingredients on all packaged products. A lot of people ask me if a certain kind of food is good for them, but when I ask them what are the ingredients in that package, they don't know. The simple truth is that you are not eating what is claimed on the front of the package, you are eating the ingredients listed on the back of that package. The companies are minimally restricted in their wording for the front of the label, but they have stricter guidelines for the official ingredient list on the back of the package. The companies are not concerned about our health; if they were, disease would be decreasing, but unfortunately, disease is on the increase. Most food companies are focused only on increasing their revenue stream and promoting healthy investment returns for shareholders—not increasing your vitality and health-wealth. We must take personal responsibility to guard our health because it affects everything we are and everything we hope to be and do.

Make time now to prepare meals at home five or six days per week to increase your health and reduce trips to the doctor. Now that you have gone around the perimeter of the grocery store and invested your time wisely in reading ingredients, below are some food preparation/cooking action items to begin taking charge of your health.

- Roast an extra chicken. You can make a stir-fry or chicken sandwiches the next day.

- Pre-wash vegetables like broccoli, celery, and carrots. Line a food container (with a top) with a paper towel to soak all the remaining water and store the vegetables in the refrigerator so they will be ready to use.
- Make double portions of spaghetti dinner. The next day serve the leftover spaghetti with stir-fry vegetables as a topping for a healthy change-up!
- Make a huge pot of vegetable soup. The leftover can be frozen in glass jars.
- Cook a whole turkey. Cut the leftovers in small pieces and freeze to use in soups.
- Make some extra fish. The leftover fish can be heated easily and served on top of a salad.
- Wash and freeze parsley in separate glass jars. Parsley does not have to thaw to be used if it's going to be cooked.
- Pre mix enough of all the spices you will use to make chili the next four or five times.
- Have fruit washed and ready to grab anytime of the day or night.
- Fill candy dishes or cookie jars with trail mix that you have made with raw nuts, raisins, dried cranberries, granola, chocolate chips, and dried fruit.

Cooking at home should be about eating "fresh," not opening cans! We have discussed tips for the grocery store experience. Now let's expand the perimeter out past the grocery store and the parking lot. Let's take a trip to the closest Farmer's Market one to two times a week. Why go to the Farmer's Market? The "fresh" fruits and vegetables at the grocery stores have been picked for days at best, and possibly for weeks, which reduces the nutritional value, taste, and texture of the food. They are picked before they are ripe to prevent spoilage while being transported throughout the country. At Farmer's Markets, the food is generally harvested the day before and possibly even the morning of market day.

Fresh fruit and vegetables have their nutrition intact, so you get the maximum benefit from your food to help your body fight and prevent disease. I see a lot of posts on finding a cure for cancer and other disease, but I don't see the emphases on eating healthy.

Battling disease isn't just about therapeutic drugs! Some people live their whole lives without drugs, but nobody can live more than a few weeks without food. Why is it so hard to believe that eating the right food is important to health? If you feel the need for the medicine, do you take just any medicine, or do you want the best medicine for your ailment? You should desire the best food for your health and reduce your chances of ever needing the medicine. We already know that there is no magic pill, yet we keep asking the doctor for that magic pill to appear from thin air.

Fresh fruit and vegetables are tastier, and if it's delicious you will eat more. Most Farmer's Markets provide only seasonal fruit and vegetables, and that is how God meant it to be. Most people today don't know what fruit and vegetables are in for each season because we have altered the availability of seasonal fruit and vegetables to every season with our modern technology, but is it as nutritious and tasty? Make it a priority to take advantage of better quality and lower prices on foods when they are in-season locally and available. Unless you live in a very special climate with constant growing seasons, there will be seasons that require you to eat frozen or dried foods; however, take advantage of fresh, in-season food as much as possible.

The shopping experience can be healthier at a Farmer's Market. Processed food is not available at the Farmer's Market, so you will not have the temptation to grab that can of beans, or minced onions in a jar. Fresh food requires preparation, and consumption within days, so the temptation of going to a fast food restaurant is decreased. Some other reasons for choosing the Farmer's Market are: Supporting your local family owned farmers by buying directly from them; they don't have the volume to compete with the food giants. By supporting your neighbors you give them the opportunity to support their families and their community. Another great reason is to protect our environment. It's been said that in the U.S. food travels an average of 1,500 miles to get to our plates. As we all know, we need to reduce the amount of natural resources we use, especially fossil fuels that are very damaging to us and to our planet. Shopping at the Farmer's Market can be psychosocially healthy because it can nurture a feeling of community as you see old friends and meet new people. The environment at the Farmer's Market is generally more cordial than a supermarket.

Start shopping with a purpose. While I was enjoying my I-pad and having a cup of organic coffee in a health-focused grocery store, I noticed the overall fitness level of the shoppers there. Shoppers across the age spectrum were agile in moving about the narrow and busy isles. The isles and shopping carts were noticeably smaller than typical large grocery chains. The scene reminded me of the grocery stores in Corinth, Greece, with the exception of the language. People in the health-focused grocery stores generally seem to exude more energy as they shop, as well as show enthusiasm during their food selection activities. It seems as if they enjoy it because they understand they are investing in their health, and they have found the investment to be returning a profit. Childhood obesity, a national epidemic, is not as apparent in stores attracting the health conscious and wellness-educated shopper.

Must you go to specialty stores to eat healthy? Most cities don't even have one; mine doesn't. You do not. There are other stores that stock healthy alternatives along with their processed foods laden with chemical additives. This is where taking charge of your health by educating yourself and purposely seeking out the best options separates you from most of the people around you. It is equally important to know what destructive choices to keep out of your cart and out of your body.

You know the saying, "You get what you pay for?" The healthier grocery stores have quality food selections with reasonable prices for the benefit they bring; that is the way it should be. It's time to expand your routine and do your food shopping in several stores for more variety of healthier options. Do not spend more time selecting a pair of shoes, or a pair of pants, than the time spent selecting food for you and your family's health. I don't see people just throwing "stuff" in their basket in the healthier grocery stores or the healthier sections of regular groceries. They stop often to read labels and compare prices with quality. They consider new seasonal food items when they appear. Get out of the rut before the rut becomes so deep you can't get out without a medical tow truck (aka ambulance). You will gain new ideas on healthier choices and healthier cooking methods just by getting out of your routine.

Grandma has traded her purse for a backpack and is fit to travel. She is walking faster than many middle age people I know. She is walking like she has a life and loves it, full of energy, nice hair, and sporting an earthy outfit. The young mother packs her baby and wears gym cloths. The shopping carts are smaller and carry more nutrition and less junk. Think of yourself as the "Special Forces" of grocery shopping and defender of your family's health. Travel light and carry only what is necessary for the mission (providing nutritious nutrients for yourself and family). Don't jeopardize the mission by carrying inferior items that don't contribute to your family's health.

CHAPTER ELEVEN

Healthy Food does not Mean Boring, Tasteless Food

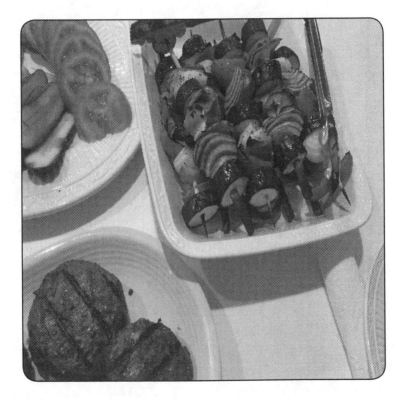

Choose well; the power of health is beautiful my friends. My husband had a conference in Nashville Tennessee, and I went with him to enjoy the beautiful hotel where he was staying and attending the conferences. He would call and check in with me when on breaks from the conference meetings. He called to tell me, proudly, that he ate a healthy lunch. The conference event provided lunch for the attendees, and this particular day there was a choice of entrée. He told me he chose a salad that consisted of spinach, avocado, which was delicious, and some lean turkey meat, which was healthy but didn't taste good because it was plain. He didn't mention all of the ingredients. He is use to my Greek cooking and knows that meat, and food in general should, be delicious and nutritious, not just nutritious. You don't have to drown your vegetables and your meat with cheese and heavy sauces to be delicious. Skip the recipes that say "cheesy " or "Mozzarella-stuffed" or "wrapped with bacon." You may be surprised how delicious real unadulterated food tastes with some simple ingredients like extra virgin olive oil, oregano, red wine vinegar, cinnamon, honey, fresh lemon juice, thyme, or turmeric. Simply nature's best will bring out the flavor of any dish, so learn how to use these ingredients.

Ancient and modern health practitioners include the use of herbs and spices to treat a variety of ailments. Greeks use herbs and spices in their cooking for flavor, aroma, and to reduce salt. Why don't we just include them now in our cooking and be ahead of the game by improving taste and increasing nutrition at the same time? We didn't have air conditioning in Lafka, and windows were always open except during the mountain winters. Walking through the narrow streets as a small girl, I could smell the aroma of what was cooking in each home. Oregano, basil, thyme, and many other herbs filled the mountain breeze with meal preparation from within each home. The herbs and spices were often so strong I wanted to go in and have dinner with them! I think you get a good appetite, or as they say in France, "bon appetite" by just smelling the food, and most of the time I knew what was cooking. I use herbs and spices in my cooking also. My next-door neighbor said one day, "You are always cooking something delicious because I can smell the aroma all the way to my house."

So add herbs and spices for a healthier life. Let's take a look at the health benefits of a few favorites.

- Oregano (Ρίγανη, pronounced REE-gah-nee). The name is a derivative of the ancient Greek word meaning, "Joy of the mountain." Greek mythology passed down over the millennia claims that Aphrodite created oregano as a symbol of happiness. Oregano has certainly made many chefs and patrons happy as they enjoyed a well-cooked, delicious Mediterranean meal. The mountains surrounding my village had plenty of oregano for anyone to pick, but you had to be fit to go up and pick it fresh. The choicest oregano grew wild, but only at the high altitudes above Lafka. I am not sure why that is. I have grown oregano in my back yard, but it doesn't have quite the same aroma as the herb from the mountain. I remember as a little girl trampling over it when we were tending to our flock of sheep because it was plentiful. Aphrodite's traditional birthplace in mythology is in Cyprus, which we visited in 2016. And, yes, Cypriots cook with a lot of oregano. Health benefits of oregano: oregano provides fiber, iron, manganese, calcium, vitamin E, and vitamin K. Oregano is also a strong anti-oxidant and has antimicrobial properties. Remember, antioxidants are recognized as natural cancer fighters. Here are a few ways to use oregano: salad dressings, salads, chili, soups, roasted chicken, stir fry, roasted potatoes, roasted root vegetables, main meat dishes, casseroles, and more. My son puts it on his eggs even. There is nothing wrong to put it on if you like the taste. Remember, food should taste good. Another health benefit is happiness per Aphrodite. You will be happy, no doubt, just knowing that you cooked something delicious and nutritious.

- Celery (Selino, Σελινο) health benefits: contains antioxidants, vitamin K, Vitamin A, folate, and potassium. Fresh celery helps protect against cancer because it contains a compound called apigenin. Apigenin has been shown effective at killing cancer cells by a mechanism called apoptosis. You can check this out yourself by searching on the National Institute of Health's website (ncbi.him. nih.gov). It has magnesium, which may help reduce blood pressure. Celery aids digestion because it provides soluble fiber. What foods can you put celery in: Stew, rice dishes, lettuce base salads, pasta salads, soups, and chili.

- Paprika (Παπρικα) made from dried and ground up sweet red peppers or chili peppers, has these health benefits: Provides Vitamin A and Vitamin C and has antibacterial properties and may help improve blood circulation. Paprika aids digestion for some individuals and is commonly believed to have anti-inflammatory properties. Paprika also contains antioxidants; antioxidants help prevent the free radicals that are commonly recognized as contributing to cancer risks. What food you can add paprika to: chicken, meatballs, potato salad, chili, risotto, couscous and more. Your taste buds will guide you to what else to try paprika in and expand your dietary options. I buy organic and recommend you consider so also.

- Cinnamon (Κανελα, pronounced kanela in Greek) – possible health benefits: A powerful antioxidant; again, antioxidants may help reduce cancer risk. Cinnamon can enhance digestion, especially the metabolism of fats. Cinnamon has anti-inflammatory properties and is thought to help fight fungal infections. Cinnamon helps lower blood sugar levels. Use caution; it is important to add cinnamon to flavor foods, like in the Greek/

Mediterranean cuisine, instead of just consuming cinnamon as a food. What foods to add cinnamon to: rice, baked apples, baked sweet potatoes, squash, roast, pastries, cakes, and more.

- Cloves (Garifalo in Greek, Γαριφαλο) - possible health benefits: aids in digestion; helps reduce the chances of cancer; clove contains Vitamins K, E, and B-6; has anti-inflammatory properties. What foods to add cloves to: use whole cloves in baked ham, beef stew, roast, or lamb. You can even spice up your tea with it. Use ground cloves in rice dishes, casseroles, chili, apple pie, pumpkin and squash dishes, and much more. Buy whole cloves and ground them yourself to ensure you are getting pure cloves and nothing else.

- Mint (dyosmos in Greek, Δυοσμο) - possible health benefits: Mint is rich in carotenes, magnesium, copper, iron, potassium, and calcium; may help prevent cancer. It may aid in digestion, calms nausea for many, and you can inhale the aroma to relieve nasal congestion. What foods to add mint to: in Greek cooking, mint is in cheese dishes, tomato based dishes, meats and rice dishes. Mint is a perennial. Mint is very easy to grow and will survive cold climates. It also adds color and aroma to flower arrangements (my sweet mother-in-law puts the mint in her flower arrangements but has never incorporated it in her cooking).

- Garlic (skordo in Greek, Σκορδο) : The Greeks would feed garlic to their athletes before they competed in the Olympic games to increase strength. Garlic's possible health benefits: reduces risk of heart disease, helps reduce the risk of cancer, has infection-fighting capability, helps reduce the risk of getting atherosclerosis; garlic has antioxidant properties, may help detoxify heavy metals in the body and possibly more. Garlic also contains manganese, vitamin B6, selenium, and vitamin C. What foods to add garlic to: roast, baked fish, meatballs, dressings, marinades, lasagna, spaghetti, and more.

- Dill (Anithos in Greek, Ανηθος) - The ancient Greeks thought of dill as a sign of wealth. Hippocrates had a recipe for a mouthwash using dill seeds. Fresh dill's possible health benefits: antioxidant properties; has calcium, manganese, copper, potassium, and magnesium. What foods to add dill to: bean soups, yogurt dip and dressing recipes, spanakopita (Greek spinach pie), breads, on salmon combined with lemon juice, on lettuce base salads, fish marinades, egg-lemon sauces, omelets, vegetables, and more.

- Turmeric (kourkoumi in Greek, Κουρκουμη) The curcumin, which is found in turmeric, provides the health benefits. I prefer turmeric instead of curcumin in my foods because it's not as pungent. Turmeric also has natural anti-inflammatory properties, may improve brain functions, and helps lower risk of heart disease. What foods to add turmeric to: potato salads, soups, smoothies, chili, sweet potatoes, roasted vegetables, rice dishes, and omelets.

- Rosemary (dendrolivano in Greek, Δενδρολιβανο) – some of the health benefits are: it may help with depression, it helps improve cognitive performance, helps with indigestion, helps improve blood circulation, has iron, calcium, and B6. What foods to add rosemary to: make a flavored olive oil, mix with butter to spread on your bread, mix in Greek yogurt, add to pot roast, roasted vegetables, and on top of salmon.

- Cilantro (koliantro in Greek, Κολιαντρο) – Toxic metal cleansing, helps prevent cardiovascular damage, a strong antioxidant, possesses anti-anxiety effects, helps improve sleep quality, has a blood sugar lowering effect, anti-bacterial and anti-fungal activity. What foods to add cilantro to: Roasted chicken with lime and cilantro recipe, guacamole, salsa, add to sour cream, rice dishes with lime or lemon juice, salad dressings, add to your coleslaw.

- Thyme (Themari in Greek, Θυμαρι) – Health benefits: strengthens the nervous system, reduces mucous in the lungs, heart healthy, helps reduce blood pressure, used in aromatherapy to boost mood, stimulates blood flow, helps prevent fungal infections, possibly helps with acne (look up tincture for additional information). What foods to add thyme to: fish dishes, grilled or roasted meats and chicken, fried potatoes in olive oil with lemon juice added instead of ketchup, broccoli soup, linguine dishes.

As you can see from the herbs above, herbs are packed with a great variety of nutritional value and health benefits. They provide important benefits such as detoxification properties, lowering blood pressure, decreasing cancer risk, helping with indigestion, providing anti-inflammatory properties, and probably benefits not identified yet. Scientists lament the loss of tropical rain forests because of the extinction of plant species before we have a chance to discover the medicinal properties of each plant. That being the case, why is it so hard for many seemingly intelligent people to believe that herbs (various plant species) can provide real health benefits? Add herbs and spices to your recipes to not only spice up your cooking and make it delicious, but to also obtain the many health benefits! Herbs are almost calorie free! Consider this, instead of making a "Detoxification Juice," why not use the herbs in your daily cooking. My Mediterranean Village Lifestyle is based on my dad's village, Lafka in the 1970's and before. Because I'm taking you back to that time period and way of life, I want to emphasize that the "Paleo" (παλαιο) or the ancient people did not take herbs and spices in a concentrated pill form. If we are going to recreate that lifestyle, we should cook with the herbs and spices and not rely on a pill for everything. That concept doesn't just apply to herbs. It is now recognized that regularly eating fish that is high in omega-3 fatty acids is superior to eating "whatever" and taking fish oil pills.

CHAPTER TWELVE

Is Organic Food Expensive?

Many people's first thought about organic foods is that they cannot possibly afford organic food or that organic foods are not worth the price. Organic foods generally cost more than the non-organic, but that doesn't necessarily mean an individual or family will have less money as a result of buying and eating organic food. Investing in Savings Bonds or an IRA will cost you money (when you invest), but we all recognize that the money invested pays us back more later in life. Organic food, along with a healthy life style that includes exercise, moderation in food and drink, and cooking at home pays back substantial interest and dividends; remember, health is the first wealth. Depending on other variables in your health and lifestyle, the payback can be pretty quick. Many individuals can pay for a whole week of organic food by simply cooking at home instead of eating out.

When you start buying better food, you may have to prioritize. Do you value cheap food and a lot of "things" in your house crammed in to full, walk-in closets, or will you value foods that nourish your body, and reduce your risk of disease? Will you continue to value the convenience of eating out, or will you choose to value home cooked meals using the healthiest ingredients. It is a lifestyle choice. It is not only choosing physical health, it is choosing family health. The family ate together in Lafka. I have friends in Cyprus, and they enjoyed family meals there also. I am not saying that you must keep your children from all activities, but if every evening is running to and fro and picking up take out or eating convenient processed foods, you are not providing your family with the opportunity of optimal health. Family is important. Don't sacrifice all family rituals (like dinner together) for every perceived opportunity for achievement. Please do not take this as an endorsement of not providing challenges and opportunities for your children; however, there must be a healthy balance!

A lot of people have their house full of "stuff." I really don't think that this is what God meant when he said in Deuteronomy 6:11 (NKJV) "...houses filled with all kinds of good things you did not provide, wells you did not dig, and vineyards and olive groves you did not plant—then when you eat and are satisfied."

When my mother died I had the task of cleaning and uncluttering the condominium to make it safe for my dad to walk around in without tripping and falling. Being in Greece and not knowing what the process was to remove large items like a broken couch, a broken table, a bed and mattress, I called a friend to ask if she knew someone that I could pay and have these items taken to the dump. To my surprise, she tells me, "Take it all outside next to the trash bin and it will be gone by morning."

I did not believe that anyone would want those broken and worn things, but as they say, "One man's trash is another man's treasure." As I was taking out the rugs and a bag of picture frames, a young man came to take them literally from my hands. The skinny non-Greek man was very polite. I felt so sorry for this young man that I actually helped him carry the stuff to his place. When we arrived, I saw a tent-like structure and that's what he called home. He told me that he needed the rugs for his kids to keep warm and clean. He needed the picture frames so he could sell them to have enough for the family to eat. That night changed my perspective on things. I have made a rule for myself, for every two items I bring in the house one item must be given away. Maybe one day I will increase it to every one item I bring in the house one must be given away. May God help us realize that stuff never makes us happy. May we realize that there are people that are hurting and in need of the very basic things like food and shelter. God tells us we should be content with having food, clothes, and shelter and that he knows our needs for tomorrow (Matthew 6:25-32).

Don't misunderstand my mother; she was a philanthropist, but because she was poor when she was young, she, like most people including me, became a slave to stuff. It's really hard to get away from buying stuff because of all the advertising gimmicks that we fall for. My recent experience with the temptation to buy stuff I didn't need was at a well-known department store. After making a purchase the sales clerk gives me a card with "store money" on it, and tells me it's worth $50, but I have to come back on another day to use it. The saying "less is more" is very true and works wonders for your budget. It is also very "liberating" as my son would say.

For many people, buying and cooking organic food may not change their budget that much at all. Many people spend a tremendous amount of money eating out. Cooking a few more meals yourself takes some time, but is much healthier and saves you enough to go a long way on your quality food purchases. And again, your family will also be emotionally healthier and able to make better decisions in life as a result of prioritizing meals at home as a family unit.

CHAPTER THIRTEEN

Olive Oil

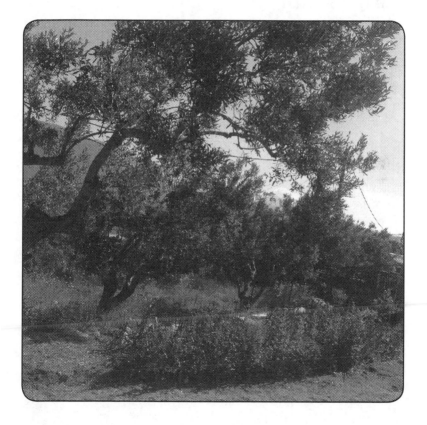

My family, like most Greek families has olive trees. My mom used olive oil in all her cooking. Olive oil is the oil of choice in the Mediterranean diet; after all, you don't see cornfields driving through the Greek countryside. It has been said that Greece has the highest olive oil intake per person in the world. We know that olive oil is good for our health because it has been used even before Christ. Deuteronomy 6:11 (NKJV) "The houses full of good things, which you did not fill, hewn-out wells which you did not dig, vineyards and olive trees which you did not plant – when you have eaten are full." Olive oil has been studied for over 50 years to examine the health benefits. It's important to use only the extra virgin olive oil and it must say, "cold pressed" on the label because they don't use a heated or chemical refined method that destroys nutrients and changes it properties. The extra virgin olive oil is extracted directly from the olive fruit by grinding the olives in thermal conditions that preserve the natural taste and health benefits. This method is called "cold pressed." It was reported on one of the news channels one morning that the newer the olive oil, the better for you. They were saying to check the expiration on your olive oil and if it's past that date, discard it and buy another newer olive oil to replace it. Are you kidding me! Why are they not using it? I go through a three-liter can of olive oil every two weeks. You can squeeze an olive and get oil out of it, unlike a soybean or a piece of corn. Below are some of the benefits of extra virgin olive oil:

- Helps reduce the risk of heart disease.
- Helps increase longevity.
- Olive oil helps satisfy your hunger (it is a good fat), which may help with weight loss.
- Helps reduce the risk of cancer.
- Helps reduce inflammation.
- Olive oil is an antioxidant.
- May help with anti–aging.
- It's rich in monounsaturated fat, which helps reduce the risk of Alzheimer's.
- Strengthens your immune system.

- Helps keep your digestive tract healthy.
- Olive oil may eventually prove to be helpful to overall bone health.
- Benefits cognitive function

How to select and store olive oil: Olive oil can become rancid, so it must be protected from light and heat. Buy extra virgin olive oil that is in dark tinted glass containers or in cans. Keep your oil in a dark cool area. I use a small stainless steel container made to pour oil from on top of my kitchen counter and store the remaining oil in the cabinet. I need to emphasize again the importance of buying only extra virgin olive oil that has "cold pressed" on the label. Labels can be misleading, as we all know by now. Example of perhaps a somewhat misleading label is "Pure olive oil." This oil can have a blend of refined and unrefined virgin olive oils. You do not want the refined olive oil because this oil has lost some of its nutrition value due to the refining process. The "refining" process does not make the oil "fine!"

I am not sure how olive trees are currently tended to in the United States. Lafka did not have olive trees because they don't thrive at the higher altitude and lower temperatures. Our olive trees were in Dervenakia (Δερβενακια), which is where we took our sheep in the winter months. It is a lower altitude and much warmer. This is where olives thrive. I never saw anyone crop-dusting olive trees. Once per year the ground around the trees was turned over and sheep and/or goat droppings were added for fertilizer. No herbicide or pesticides were used. Sheep and goats helped keep weeds down to an acceptable level. Olive trees also grew wild in many places. My father would often graft branches from cultivated trees onto wild trees so the wild tree would produce a higher quality olive. Grafting onto the tree with an established root system produced good olives quicker than planting a new tree. You can buy organic olive oil in the United States. The oil we last purchased was organic and was very good quality. I do not think it is as necessary to buy organic olive oil as it is to buy cold-pressed, extra virgin.

CHAPTER FOURTEEN

Red Meat, Sugar, and Salt Consumption in the Village

"It is far more important to know what person the disease has than what disease the person has." -Hippocrates

Most families in Lafka ate red meat about once per week. For most families this was on Sunday, and it was served as more like a side-portion. The meal was still predominately vegetables, legumes, and homemade bread. My American husband will never forget the first time he went to Greece and my sister had us over to her house for dinner. When it was time to eat, she placed a plate full of fresh green beans cooked in olive oil and tomatoes in front of every one. Then she took the roasted leg of goat and placed it in the middle of the table. My husband looked at me and asked in shock, "Is this plate of green beans all for me?" Red meat consumption is something that modern medicine and natural nutritionists agree on. A lot of red meat is not good for you.

Sodium intake should also be limited. Salt is a good seasoning and a necessary electrolyte, but is used excessively in processed foods and most restaurant food. Excessive intake of sodium can contribute to high blood pressure, and high blood pressure contributes to heart disease and stroke risk, as well as renal failure. Salt causes the kidneys to excrete less water. The extra water increases the blood pressure. Over time, the increased blood pressure causes the inner walls of the artery to become thicker, which makes the inside diameter smaller; this only limits blood flow to vital organs and increases blood pressure further. You would be surprised to know that a lot of the salt in your diet is found in processed foods such as soups, cold cuts, canned foods, and breakfast cereals. It is a good idea to check the sodium on the back of the label before you buy processed food. It is wise to eliminate all processed foods, and cook at home to control what goes in your food. It is recommended to eat less than 2,300 mg (2,300 mg of salt = 1 teaspoon) per day. In Lafka people used a lot of vinegar, fresh lemon juice, and lots of herbs to give food flavor, which cuts down the need for a lot of salt. Salt should be iodized, and it should not contain dextrose.

The human body cannot function without sodium (salt). Salt is necessary for nerve conduction and for muscle contractions. Loss of sodium through excessive sweating often causes muscle cramps. My 97-year old father, Yianni, had salt eliminated from his diet for several months out of concern for his blood pressure. Shortly after that he began to complain of chronic and severe headaches, as well as leg pain that kept him from being able to walk to his coffee shop. He visited a different physician who determined that he was hyponatremic (low in sodium). Salt should have been left in his diet, but used in moderation. After adding some salt back into his diet, his headaches stopped and his muscle pain left. Part of the problem was his caregiver tried to keep his blood pressure as low as a 20 or 30 year old. It is now recognized by most doctors that the elderly will have some elevation in blood pressure and it is not necessary to treat it. You should discuss what is acceptable with your doctor, but the normal less than 120 systolic may not be realistic for many people at an advanced age.

Sugar is another pervasive insult to our health. Medical research is starting to acknowledge what natural nutritionists have said for some time about sugar. And that is that sugar adversely affects many physiological systems. Sugar has adverse effects on the nervous system and is thought to be a prime suspect in the development of Alzheimer's disease because sugar fuels inflammation; chronic inflammation is not good. It is not an accident that Alzheimer Disease has increased at an alarming rate in our generation. There is more discussion now about sugar causing inflammation in the circulatory system with the result of increased plaque formation. Plaque on the inner layer of arteries is what causes most heart attacks and strokes. Mainstream medicine still focuses on cholesterol when discussing cardiovascular disease, but I think that will change over the next decade or so. Currently the use of "statin" drugs to lower cholesterol is very profitable for the pharmaceutical companies. The same inflammation can cause poor circulation in the extremities. We have also known that diabetics are at a significantly greater risk for vascular disease affecting most vital organ systems (heart, brain, kidneys etc.). Diabetes is the leading cause of foot and leg amputations, and of course we all know that inadequate processing of sugar in the body is the evil brought on by diabetes.

Using sugar, white flour, and any foods made with these ingredients did not happen in Lafka or Dervenaki when I left Greece to begin my new life in America. The only oil used was extra virgin olive oil for everything from baking, to frying, and on salads. Olive oil helps reduce bad LDL cholesterol and increase good HDL cholesterol and keeps your arteries supple. In the Greek Orthodox denomination it is customary to fast two days a week and fast 40 days before Easter. You don't have to be a Greek Orthodox to incorporate fasting in to your diet. You can fast for spiritual or health reasons. Fasting can help the body detoxify, and there are several types of fasting. My favorite, which I recommend, is to give up meat of any kind two days a week. Most people in the village had walnut trees. Walnuts are a good source of omega-3 fatty acids. It has been said that walnuts can reduce the risk of heart disease by 8 to 10 %. Staying active is a huge component of heart health and the norm in Lafka.

Staying active supported healthy physiological functioning for the residents of Lafka because our bodies are made for activity; they are not made to be sedentary. Activity improves the efficiency of the lymphatic system and the cardiovascular system. Activity is also key in the prevention of obesity. Obesity was very rare when I left Greece. Obesity is an epidemic in America and other countries where the modern western diet has emerged. Obesity has had devastating effects on our cardiovascular system (as well as other systems).

Stress-management is important to keeping the heart healthy. When you are stressed the blood vessels become constricted and the heart is forced to work harder at pumping in order to circulate the blood throughout the body adequately. It seems ironic that often the more God blesses us with "success" in life, the more we find to stress-out about. Maybe that is why he tells us in the Sermon on the Mount not to worry about tomorrow!

Extra virgin olive oil should be the only oil in your house, with the exception of oil for your lawnmower, which you should push and not ride. Olive oil is rich in monounsaturated fats, and olive oil is now commonly known to reduce the risk of heart disease. I have said this before, but I want to make sure you get this: In my village, Lafka, olive oil was the only oil used! The Mediterranean diet has been studied over and over and olive oil remains the oil of choice for health. Switching to olive oil even later in life is beneficial.

CHAPTER FIFTEEN

Minimal Processing

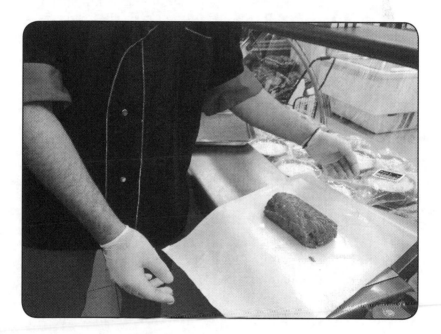

Do you really know what fresh meat looks like? What does minimal processing actually mean and why should you care?

Do you remember ever hearing of a recall involving a side of beef or a whole, unprocessed chicken? Probably not! The majority of the recalled meat is processed; it is either cut-up and packaged in pieces or ground. You will not watch the news very many days before hearing of another recall of meat contaminated with either

Salmonella or E-Coli bacteria. Processed meat has also made the news recently when questions arose about the integrity of the labeling. Specifically, was the beef really 100% beef? The most prevalent questions are about ground meat.

Does "Pink Slime" sound like a healthy nutrient to you? Would you order it as a hamburger topping like you would tomato and onion? Pink slime is made from trimmings processed with heat to separate components, sprayed with ammonia to kill bacteria, and shipped to supermarkets to be added to meat—it is pink in color. Discussion about the use of this product continues at the time of this writing. My opinion is that the less food is processed, the better it is. In my opinion, "Pink Slime" is an overly processed product!

What is minimal processing? We know that if it has more than one ingredient it has been processed, but what if it's only one ingredient, for example, chicken breast, chicken legs, ground beef, or stew meat pieces? The less the meat is handled, the lower the risk of contamination. In Greece you have the option to this day of going to the butcher shop and selecting a cut of beef and asking the butcher to ground it for you in front of your eyes. You also have the option of selecting a chicken and asking the butcher to cut it in pieces for you. Most Greeks take that option, but in America if you ask a butcher to do that, he/she will do it but is not customary, so most people don't take that option or even realize it is an option.

Buy what you will need for the next two to three days. Greeks go the markets multiple times each week to ensure fresh items in the kitchen. In fact, Europeans in general tend to have much smaller refrigerators. It may be convenient to buy the meat and freeze it, but you don't know if the meat is not spoiled unless you open it before you freeze it. It's possible not to notice it's spoiled after thawing because the meat may be partially frozen when you start the cooking process. When I stopped freezing my meat and started using only fresh meat, I noticed that on several occasions I had bought spoiled chicken and had to take it back.

Below are suggestions to reduce contamination:

- Buy a whole chicken instead of chicken parts and cut it in pieces yourself. Your mother or grandmother will be more than glad to show you how, or go to the Internet and watch a video on how to cut up a chicken. God made a chicken with dark and white meat, and He is the omniscient God. Dark meat has some benefits that white meat does not, and the white meat has some benefits that the dark meat does not have; so eat them both. White meat is lower in fat and a good source of protein without extra fat. Red meat contains more fat, but also contains more vitamins and minerals. Dark chicken meat contains: "iron, zinc, selenium, as well as vitamins A, K and the B complex – B1 (thiamine), B2 (riboflavin), B3 (niacin) B6, B9 (folate) and B12 (cobalamin).

- Select a cut of beef from the meat department and ask the butcher to grind it for you or buy a meat grinder and do it yourself. My good friend used to say to me, "How do you know that the already ground up meat does not include nose, ears, tail…." He had me grinding my own meat in the 80's. He had grown use to living by himself and worked on an assembly line at a tobacco factory. He told me his job was hard and his cloths were soaked with sweat from spring to fall. He did not have anyone at home to cook, clean, or go to the market. He did not even have a dishwasher, but he did not compromise when it came to eating healthy food. With convenience you usually take a greater risk with yours and your family's health!

"We write our own destiny; we become what we do." Madame Chiang Kai-Shek

CHAPTER SIXTEEN

Healthy Solutions to a Healthy Weight

Dieting does not lead to a healthy maintained weight for most people, and it does not lead to a healthy lifestyle. It has been said that most people gain their weight back plus more when they stop their diet. Processed "diet foods" with little or no nutritional value and questionable ingredients may increase health problems.

Most people are confused about what actually are healthy foods that could aid loosing weight due to so many deceptions on the front of the labels such as, low-fat, sugar-free, fat-free, or lite to name a few. The ingredients are listed on the back of the label; it's up to us to decide if we are going to take the time to read the information or not. I personally believe that the responsibility is on the consumer to determine if the food is healthy or not, and that can easily be determined by the ingredients. It's the actual ingredients that we are eating and not the marketing adjectives on the front of the package.

The corporations are not looking out for you; they are looking at the financial bottom line. Profits are what stockholders are looking for. All these marketing deceptions have cost Americans their health. We need to dig deeper in to the diet foods to see what is actually going into our bodies. What are you really eating when you consume diet foods? Let's take a look at some diet foods and their ingredients:

- Fat-free" Half & Half ingredients: skim milk, corn syrup, carrageenan, sodium citrate, dipotasium phosphate, mono and diglycerides, vitamin A palmitate, color added (the type of color added is not listed, how convenient).
- Sugar-free" Apricot Preserves: water, polydextrose, maltodextrin, fruit pectin, citric acid, locust bean gum, natural flavor, potassium sorbate, sucralose, calcium chloride, yellow #5, yellow #6.
- Lite" Ranch dressing ingredients: water, soybean oil, maltodextrin, distilled vinegar, buttermilk powder, sugar, corn syrup, modified corn starch, salt, Contains 2% or less of each of the following: phosphoric acid, color added, onion powder, garlic powder, xanthan gum, monosodium glutamate, egg yolk, sorbic acid, and sodium benzonate, and calcium disodium EDTA, lemon juice concentrate, propylene glycol, algnate, spices, natural flavor (milk), disodium inosinate, disodium guanylate, DL tocopheryl, (vitamin E), soy lecithin.
- Light" butter ingredients: water, butter, canola oil, buttermilk, contains less than 2% of food starch-modified, tapioca maltodextrin, salt, distilled monoglycerides, lactic acid, potassium sorbate, sodium benzoate, natural flavor, xanthan gum, PGPR, and beta-carotene.

The "diet" foods leave out nutrition that our body needs and that helps satisfy our hunger naturally; you end up eating more chemicals and non-nutritious food because the body isn't satisfied. Don't be fooled into obesity! There are more fat-free food choices than ever; however, obesity is claiming more Americans than ever before. Fat-free and sugar-free doesn't work.

Don't go on another fad diet, instead set out on the road to success by learning how to make healthy choices that result in lost pounds. As a bonus you will live a happier, healthier, and longer life. Eating healthy does not necessarily mean eating less or eating "diet" foods. Eating healthy is simply changing from food that is man made to food that was created by God. God created you, and He also created the food that you should be eating to maintain health, which includes a healthy weight. Who are you going to trust with your health, God or big food companies?

Here are some tips on the best and healthiest way to lose weight and keep it off:

- Eliminate processed foods. Eat foods that are close to their natural source. Processed foods are full of additives, and have very little nutrition. Your body craves nutrition, so you continue to be hungry even though you already had a meal.
- Eliminate all canned foods, and instead buy either fresh or frozen. Be sure to read the ingredients in the frozen foods. For example, if you are buying frozen peas, the ingredients should be peas.
- Eliminate all sugar, including sugar substitutes. There are over 40 different names of sugar so please read the ingredients in everything you buy. Use a little raw honey, pure maple syrup or pure stevia for sweeteners. Take the ten-day challenge to eliminate sugar and all of its forms listed below:
  - Barley malt
  - Brown sugar
  - Cane sugar
  - Carob syrup
  - Corn syrup
  - Corn syrup solids

- Dextran
- Dextrose
- Diatase
- Diastatic malt
- Ethyl maltol
- Fructose
- Glucose
- High-fructose corn syrup
- Lactose
- Malt syrup
- Maltodextrin
- Maltose
- Mannitol
- Molasses
- Refiner's syrup
- Sorbitol
- Sorghum syrup
- Sucrose
- Sugar
- Turbinado sugar

- Eat an organic apple with the skin every morning with your breakfast. Apples are a great way to stay regular because of the high fiber; additionally it helps stabilize blood-sugar levels, and may help lower blood cholesterol.
- Use it or lose it! Walk 5-7 times a week (outdoors if weather permits). Walking will not cost you anything, and the benefits are amazing. Walking helps you lose weight and keep it off, strengthens your heart, and reduces your risk of type 2 diabetes. Walking outdoors helps prevent dementia. Walking counts as a weight-bearing exercise, so it decreases your chances of getting osteoporosis, and tones your body. Walking outside in daylight provides your vitamin D, gives you energy, and improves your mood.

- Drink six to eight glasses of purified water (not in plastic bottles) every day to flush out toxins, help with digestion, improve your skin, lubricate joints, and regulate body temperature. Water also helps you lose weight by replacing all other drinks that may have sugar or sugar substitute.
- Dine out once a week as a celebration, but don't gorge. Dining out should be looked at as enjoying the company and the atmosphere, as well as not having to cook or do the dishes.
- Go nuts! Eat raw walnuts, and almonds (roast the almonds first) several times a week in salads, yogurt, fruit salads, oatmeal, stir fry, and anything else you would like them in. Some of the benefits: helps control weight, contains omega-3, provides powerful antioxidants, helps reduce the risk of cancer, is rich in vitamin E, provides natural fiber, magnesium, and more. Nuts contain healthy fats that help satisfy your hunger even in a small quantity like a handful.
- Exercise 3-4 times a week. Start out slow, and if you are under a physician's care, please discuss your exercise plans with your physician first. Exercise increases your metabolism, which will cause you to burn calories even when you are doing nothing.
- Cut down on red meat, which is high in saturated fat, which may prevent you from losing those extra pounds. In addition, most research shows that too much red meat may shorten lifespan. Cholesterol has been considered the chief culprit in cardiovascular disease for decades now, but there is newer evidence that indicates that it is not actually the cholesterol that is to blame, but the saturated animal fat.
- Eat saltwater fish including wild-caught salmon often. Note: read the ingredients, the only ingredient listed should be the fish name.

- Take the trash (cookies, ice cream, donuts, chips etc.) out of the house. Replace them with fresh and frozen fruit, raw nuts, 70% cocoa and above chocolate bars, regular Greek yogurt.
- Eliminate all white flour out of your diet. White flour makes you fat, contributes to constipation, and clogs your digestive system.
- Do a liver cleanse. The best liver cleanse I know is fresh lemon juice and water in the morning 30 minutes before breakfast. A liver-cleanse benefits the overall function of the important organ. Below are some of the functions of the liver:
  - Controlling levels of fats, amino acids and glucose in the blood
  - Combating infections in the body
  - Clearing the blood of particles and infections including bacteria
  - Neutralizing and destroying drugs and toxins
  - Manufacturing bile
  - Breaking down food and turning it into energy
  - Manufacturing, breaking down and regulating numerous hormones including sex hormones"
- For a week, commit to cleanse your liver every morning before breakfast. Get a bag of lemons and let's get it done!
- Fast - The Greek Orthodox Church believes that fasting helps heal the afflictions of the body and spirit. The Daniel fast (Daniel 10:2-3) has become the favorite fast method for many protestant church members. I personally prefer the Daniel fast. There are two Daniel fasts that people practice. The first fast encourages people to eat only vegetables, and drink only water. The second fast encourages people to give up meat, wine, and rich foods for a period of time. You can choose to fast once a week, two times a week or even two times a year for a period of

40 days like the Greek Orthodox and Catholic churches. Whatever works for you, but if you are under a doctor's care you must discuss this with your doctor before fasting.

- -Do not eat after six p.m. or 3-4 hours before bedtime. Have fresh fruit if you need something before going to bed.

If you are under a doctor's care, have health issues, or are taking medication, you must consult with your doctor before making any changes to your diet.

CHAPTER SEVENTEEN

Colon Health

Colon cancer is the second leading cancer killer in America!

I don't understand why people would put themselves through a colonoscopy exam but are unwilling to change their lifestyle? A colonoscopy will not cure cancer, but it may detect colon cancer in earlier stages. A healthy diet along with exercise will substantially reduce the risk of developing colon cancer. Colon cancer is the second leading cancer killer in American; only lung cancer kills more. And just as we know that smoking is responsible for the majority of lung cancer deaths, we now know that what we eat is primarily responsible for the development of colon cancer. I am not suggesting that you disregard your doctor's orders for a colonoscopy; I am suggesting that you should focus on what to do to prevent colon cancer. Instead of waiting until the next colonoscopy to see if you have cancer, get serious about disease prevention by educating yourself and being willing to make simple changes in your diet and lifestyle!

There are many signs of an unhealthy colon. The most common sign is chronic constipation. A healthy person should have at least one bowel movement per day. Elimination should be complete, easy, and fast. Some other possible signs are a potbelly, excessive gas, bloating, and feeling tired or being mentally foggy. Blood in your stool is a sign that should be taken seriously. If you have blood in your stool (can be red or can be a black, tarry stool) you should see a doctor for evaluation without delay.

Fiber is one of the most important elements of colon health. The National Cancer Institute recommends, "consuming 20-30 grams of fiber a day." Fiber is needed to keep bowels moving freely and to help break down and remove any existing build-up. Think of fiber as a sponge that absorbs toxins and sweeps them out of your system. Decreasing the amount of time waste stays in your body reduces the chances of getting colon cancer. Lafka's people ate a diet full of fiber-rich foods such as lentils, northern beans, black eye peas, whole wheat bread, whole-wheat pasta, and fresh vegetables from their gardens, nuts, and seasonal fruits. I remember my mom baking bread in the clay oven outside. I remember the wonderful aroma of fresh baked bread. My parents, as well as all of the people in Lafka, raised their own wheat. Take out that trash (white flour products of any kind); it's your first step to a healthy colon. At the end of this section is a list of foods that are high in fiber.

Here are some other things you can do to reduce your risk of colon cancer and achieve and maintain a healthy colon:

- Get out in the sun 15-20 minutes per day to make vitamin D by sunrays. Adequate amounts of Vitamin D help reduce the chances of colon cancer. If it's sunny, you can benefit even when it's cold outside and even when there is snow on the ground! Bundle up and go for a short walk to get vitamin D from the sun, and you will get exercise as a bonus. Princess, my precious mixed-breed, canine best friend that we adopted from the animal shelter, will keep reminding me that we need to go for a walk until we get it done. Being outdoors early in the morning with the rooster until around 11 am was the lifestyle in Lafka. There was a lot of required outdoor activity such as cultivating the fields, working in family gardens, tending to sheep flocks, and feeding the chickens. Also, late afternoon, after lunch and a nap, everyone got back out to finish the daily work.

- Exercise three or four times a week (talk to your doctor before starting an exercise program). Physical activity is a must if you want to be healthy. Physical activity isn't just for weight management; many body systems, including the digestive system, require physical activity to work effectively. Yianni, and all the people in Lafka, performed physical activity just by doing the daily work. Lafka did not have a gym, and it did not have any modern conveniences. Physical activity was required from the time they were able to walk to the time God called them home.
- Drink plenty of water. You should drink 6 or more glasses of water each day. Water is important for many body systems, but is especially important to keep the bowels working effectively and on a regular schedule.

High fiber foods list:

Raspberries- 8 grams
Blackberries – 7.6 grams
½ Avocado – 6.7 grams
Pears – 5.5 grams
Apples w/skin – 3 – 4 grams
Bananas – 3 grams
Oranges – 3-4 grams
Navy beans – 19 grams
White beans – 19 grams
Kidney beans – 15.6 grams
Lentils – 15.6 grams

Pinto beans – 15 grams
Black beans – 15 grams
Lima beans – 13.2 grams
Acorn squash – 9 grams
Peas – 8.8 grams
Raw spinach – 7 grams
Carrots – 5.2 grams
Broccoli – 5.1 grams
Cauliflower – 5 grams
Bran flakes – 7 grams
Whole wheat pasta – 6.3 grams
Almonds – 4.2 grams

CHAPTER EIGHTEEN

What are You Doing After a Serious Illness?

This is a critical question to ask? What am I going to do to improve my health and help my body recover? What am I doing different in my lifestyle since I am in remission from cancer? I asked this question to all the people I know that are, or were, battling a disease, and 95% of the time the answer is "I am not doing anything different" or "back to normal life." You have heard people say that eating better, taking supplements, and exercise are not going to make a difference. Ask yourself this question, "If I have the same lifestyle as before the disease, why do I expect my body to fight it and keep me healthy now?" It's like the quote I read long ago that says, "Insanity is doing the same thing over and over and expecting different results." Your body needs your help to get to a better state to fight disease, and the way it gets to a better state is being provided with good, clean, non-processed foods, a house clean of toxins, regular exercise, and meditation on God's Word to reduce stress and be spiritually healthy. The responsibility for your health is yours, not the doctor's or the pharmaceutical companies. The sooner you realize this and start taking control of your own health destiny, the sooner you will be building your road to better health.

The air you breath is also important to your health and should also be a consideration during and after an illness (best would be to have done this before illness). When was the last time you took your comforters, sofa throws, blankets, or pillows outside? My mom used to take the blankets and comforters outside every week during dry sunny days, to shake them and drape them over the rails of the veranda. She would also take all of the rugs outside to give them a good beating with a broom so the dust and dirt would be removed. She was concerned about indoor pollution even in our way-less-than-airtight home! We also had no indoor animals.

Today our homes are generally more airtight, which makes them better for heating and cooling, but horrible for eliminating indoor pollution. Studies show that in all but the most terrible cities, indoor air is more polluted than outside air. Fresh air does a home good, which does your body good also. There are benefits to practicing the "Vasiliki" (my mother) method. If you have pets, don't forget the pet bedding; they should also go outside for a good shaking and fresh air ventilation. The shaking of comforters, blankets, rugs, etc. removes dust, which is also food for dust mites because the majority of the dust is from dead skin cells. Pets shed a lot of hair and dander, and shaking bedding outside removes them from your house. You can also place pillows, children's toys, and dog toys in the freezer for 24 hours to kill the mites. If you don't have a big enough freezer to put big items in, take them outside when the temperature is below freezing, but protect them from rain or snow. Removing dust may improve allergies and asthma. I read this tip you can use if you have pets; run a wet cloth over the pet's fur each day.

You should make it a point to open the windows at regular intervals throughout the week (how long to keep them open will depend on the weather), especially the bedroom windows where we spend eight hours (sleep is important too) a day. Be sure to open more than one window for cross ventilation. If you or a family member suffers from asthma or allergies, you should probably open the windows at night when the air-born allergen count is lower. Reducing the level of indoor pollutants may benefit even those with allergies to natural outdoor pollens because chronic sinus or respiratory inflammation may increase your inflammatory reaction to other substances.

Other types of indoor pollutions include household cleaners. Consider buying non-toxic, environmentally friendly cleaning products for your home. There are now some great product selections to choose from to protect your health and your family's health. Some of the warnings on the brand name toxic products are very scary if you take the time to read them. One example is on a bleach flushing tablet; "Hazardous to humans and pets," "If inhaled move person to fresh air," and "Note to physicians: probable mucosal damage may contraindicate the use of gastric lavage." I don't think I want that in my house; it sounds more like a "do not enter, hazardous material."

Common types of indoor pollution include: Molds, scented candles, air fresheners, burning of wood, new carpet, products made with polyvinyl chloride, glues and adhesives, paint, pressed-wood products, upholstered furniture, radon, secondhand smoke, lead particles widely used in house paint until it was banned in 1978, and asbestos. Are you ready to open up your windows now for some real fresh air? I'm gasping for air by just reading all these facts.

Some of the symptoms of indoor pollution include watery eyes, runny nose, sneezing, itching, dizziness, fatigue, coughing, and headache.

CHAPTER NINETEEN

Happy and Healthy

It is the simple things in life that make us happy, and healthy!

My son and his lovely wife recently moved to Chattanooga, Tennessee. Chattanooga is a beautiful city surrounded by beautiful and historic mountains. The street and the neighborhood where they live have a lot of construction going on. This neighborhood appears to be the revival of the older city with new construction and remodeling of older homes in progress around most every corner. As I had my coffee each morning in their dining area with an elevated view, I noticed that the construction workers across the street had a fire going and were playing Hispanic music on the radio. They took their breaks around the fire, which they built every chilly morning with scraps of wood from the building site. Now I have a better understanding of what my son was telling me on the phone before I came to visit. Only he thought that the guys were burning the wood because they wanted to get rid of the scrap wood instead of taking it to the dumpsite. He also was concerned that the fire may get out of control and spread.

What I saw was the workers trying to stay warm as they got the day going. Construction workers are known to start early, and it was still winter at the time. They used the available natural material, probably like they were accustomed to in their home country. A "campfire" provides warmth, but it also brings people together for a common experience. The construction workers played their favorite music to connect them to happy memories of home and family. I am Greek and I feel connected to my homeland when I hear Greek music.

The friendly workers were always ready to greet the neighbors with a good morning and happily continue their work. They all seemed to enjoy the small fire and the music; it was a small thing that made them happy. Engaging in activities with those that we share values and experiences with is one way to foster happiness in our lives. Happiness is a critical part of health we cannot leave out. Happiness contributes to good health, but good health should also contribute to happiness. Material goods do not bring us genuine happiness! Valuing the basic needs and blessings of life bring happiness. You can see this with children. A child with a room full of toys is usually quickly bored. The child would rather have mom or dad engaging in a simple game with them. Years later, both the child and the parents will remember and value the time spent playing—long after the pile of toys in the floor are pitched and forgotten.

It is becoming more and more clear that our thoughts can contribute to our health or harm or limit our health. Being in a good mood benefits our blood pressure, boosts our immune system, and improves mental function. Stress is known to contribute to illness, and stress and unhappiness are often woven together.

"Rejoice in the Lord always. Again I will say rejoice!" Philippians 4:4 (NKJV)

Here are some simple suggestions to be happier:

- Start the day with a simple, "Thank you God;" after all, he is the one that gives us each new day.

- Write a scripture verse or a positive quote on a sticky note and post it on the bathroom mirror. Change the post every week.
- Take a walk outdoors in the fresh air as often as possible.
- Get 15–30 minutes of sunshine often, before 10 a.m., or after 4 p.m. Even in cold weather we should allow the sun to shine on us
- Listen to Christian music; this is very uplifting.
- Take a group exercise class.
- Go on a picnic.
- Limit time spent with negative people.
- Schedule something fun on a regular basis. Everyone needs something to look forward to. Half of the fun is the planning and anticipation. If you are always busy fun won't happen unless you schedule it.
- Perform an act of kindness, and it does not have to be money. For example, my widowed neighbor is a private person and has been as long as I have known her. On occasion I take a jar of homemade soup and homemade bread and leave it on the table outside. When I get home, I call her to let her know it's out there. It makes me feel good that I did something for someone else that day and it lets her know she is not forgotten.
- Eat healthy. You knew I was going to implement this one, but it's only because I care. Healthy food not only reduces the chances of us getting disease it will give us the nutrition the brain needs to sustain happiness. If you are not eating healthy food, you are eating unhealthy food -- just saying.
- Don't repost or hit "like" on quotes that are negative when you are on social media. I see so many people doing this, which is not helping them, but it's actually working against their own happiness. If your friends on social media are posting things that upset you, hide their stuff.

You don't have to un-friend them, but you don't have to wallow in negativity either.

"May the God of hope fill you with all joy and peace as you trust in him, so that you may overflow with hope by the power of the Holy Sprit." Romans 15:13

CHAPTER TWENTY

Animal Therapy

A Dog is a man's best friend, but can also be his healer! This is not a Mediterranean Greek Village practice, but it can be a valuable part of a healthy life that I am throwing in anyway!

Growing up in Greece until I was eleven, the thought of having a dog in the house was unheard of. People had hunting dogs, watchdogs, and sheep dogs in Lafka. Dogs were considered unclean in the house. Cats were allowed in the house only because they kept the mice out. I don't remember people petting dogs or cats for their affection or for therapeutic reasons. I will never forget the time when my dad, 92 years old at the time, decided to come to the United States alone to have his gallbladder removed. He had been told in Athens that he was too old and it's not worth the risk of surgery. Of course, they neglected to tell him that a septic gallbladder would cause death, which is quite a risk. Little did they know that my dad had a determination that not only was he going to live through this, he was doing it without chronic pain.

Our cat, Panther, loved to sleep by dad's head every night after surgery. For some odd reason dad allowed Panther to sleep with him even though he would have not entertained it when I was a little girl. Little did dad know that Panther actually provided him with comfort, reduced his blood pressure, relieved his depression from being away from his home, and improved his mood.

We also have a rescued dog named Princess. Let's just say that dad was not very friendly towards our dog being in the house, and Princess knew that he did not want her in the house so she kept her distance. Princess is my personal fitness instructor. Princess demands to go for a walk every day. She is a big dog and needs her exercise. I think she looks forward to sniffing all the scents from other dogs along the way, which necessitates me making frequent stops along the way. Princess reminds me that walking requires the senses of, smell, touch, sight, and sound. Dogs are routine animals, and they will remind you if you haven't taken them for their walk. My dog's way of reminding me is by looking at me with those sad puppy eyes and walking towards the closet where I keep my tennis shoes. It's still an enigma to me how she knows the difference between we are going for a walk, and I'm going to the gym when I put my tennis shoes on.

It's easy to forget that those walks are helping us too. A daily walk is one of the best exercises you can do and it does not cost anything. Playing tug-of-war with the dog because it saw an animal and wants to chase it is a great exercise for the arms too. As you walk, when your mind wanders, and it will, bring yourself back to the moment to enjoy the sights and smells of the outdoors. You will also get lots of vitamin D on those sunny days to help prevent cancer, and osteoporosis. Everyone may not be able to or want to have a pet because of work schedules or certain health issues; however, there is much benefit to be gained from pets.

Pets enrich our lives by keeping us physically active and fit. Dogs, especially medium to large dogs, need to be walked daily. A dog will motivate us to move because they are routine animals, and they will remind us with that sad look "it's time to take me for a walk." They need to be fed two to three times a day and taken outside to use the bathroom, which requires getting off that couch or the easy chair several times a day whether we feel like it or not; they train us to move. They need play time. My dog will bring us her ball and growl in a playful way for us to engage in the activity. She also likes to play chase with my husband. Everyday when my husband gets home, she growls playfully and backs up to the back door to let him know it's time to go out and play chase. It's hard to not participate with her because she is so adorable as we all think our pets are. No matter how tired he is he feels guilty not playing with her.

Pets can help us fight depression. Dogs, and cats are entertaining, which allows us to escape from our issues. Our dog Princess will lay on her back with belly up ready for a belly rub, or she will bring her ball so we can play throw and catch, or she will look me in the eyes with that sweet look when she wants to go out and bark at the neighbor's dog again for the fiftieth time in one day! They are great companions. Having our pet keeps us from feeling alone. I read a quote that helps describe why dogs in particular help us with depression: "A dog will teach you unconditional love. If you can have that in your life, things won't be too bad." -Robert Wagner- (actor)

Pets also help us reduce our stress level. Have you noticed that even if you are petting a friend's dog or cat it is calming? Pets warm our hearts because they provide love and acceptance. They make us smile and laugh with their amusing and loveable actions. Cats and dogs greet their owner at the door with love and affection. Dogs, and cats have the natural tendency to be social. We are so drawn to their cute activity that we forget our problems and relax. Less stress means a longer, healthier life.

I strongly recommend that you get your pet from an animal shelter. My daughter taught us the importance of rescuing an animal. She has a dog she rescued from the animal shelter. She rescued a kitten hiding in a bush close to where she was working as a lifeguard. She also rescued our dog Princess when she and her dad went to a pet store to get dog food for her dog. Rescued cats and dogs make us feel good because we saved their lives, but the animal can also rescue us by adding meaning to our lives, adding years to our lives, and adding joy to our lives

CHAPTER TWENTY-ONE

Give, and it will be Given Unto You

"Give, and it will be given to you. A good measure, pressed down, shaken together and running over, will be poured into your lap. For with the measure you use, it will be measured to you." Luke 6:38 (NKJV)

Yianni, my dad, shared some amazing stories about how he gave out of his heart to very needy people. I will share with you three stories, one of which I saw with my own eyes.

Yianni was a young man in his early twenties watching his flock of sheep in the hills of Dervenaki, Greece during the depression. One day when he finished milking his sheep, a man, his young wife and their very young child approached my dad. After greeting dad, they asked if he was going to make feta cheese, and if so they would wait and take the whey protein, which is the by-product of cheese production. They were humble and did not want to ask dad for milk because they could see that dad was a poor "Tsopane" shepherd. Dad was so compassionate that he grabbed the bucket of fresh milk and filled their container. After hugging dad and saying thank you they continued their journey. Other people noticed that the couple were carrying a milk jug so they also stopped. Dad filled several containers as people kept coming up to beg for milk. After the people stopped coming he continued with making the cheese. When the process was finished, he had the regular amount of cheese made even though he started with significantly less milk.

The second story is from 1941, and Greece was suffering from depression. The Greeks called it "The 41," and it is understood that it was the worst depression they had ever experienced. This was a time when people went hungry and as Dad stated in his memoirs, it was much worse in the cities. My dad was 24 years old in 1941 and was a shepherd, spending most of his days with his flock of sheep. The story I'm going to translate to you is from my dad's memoirs, and I picked this one also because it will help us make the connection between real, God-created food and health.

Dad had his sheep at one of the family's small farmlands close to one of the small villages called Κοντοσταβλοσ (Kondostavlos). Occasionally he would go into the village to have his Greek coffee and meet up with the local friends. On one day when he was at the village, a young girl was walking next to the coffee shop, and he noticed that she was crying. So he went up to her and asked why she was crying? The young girl said that her younger sister was very sick, and she went on to explain that her uncle took her sister to the hospital in Corinth. The doctor at the hospital told him that her sister's liver was diseased and gave her medicine to take. The doctor explained that if she did not take it daily she would die. The doctor had also told her that if she didn't eat enough she would die.

Dad thought, "I don't have much," but he felt sorry for her and her family so he told her to go home and tell her parents that they can bring her to the tent (where dad slept to be close to his sheep). He told her that he would feed her sister plenty of fresh yogurt, feta cheese, sheep milk, and olives, which was all that my dad had. Dad happened to be drinking coffee that day with one of his friends, which owned a mill very close to the village (talking about God's timing). He told dad that he would go right away and bring bread and he would provide all the bread needed. Dad had a close friend near him that also was a young shepherd, and Dad shared the situation with his friend when he went back to the flock.

The little girl went home and told her parents what dad had said, and the parents were so happy because they were very poor and dad could feed her better than they could. The parents put their little sick girl on a mule, packed her medicine, and took her to dad that evening. With tearful eyes they thanked dad and gave him hugs. Dad gave her parent's feta cheese and yogurt to take back to the other children. The next day Dad's friend that had the mill brought them a fresh cooked chicken, and about ten boiled eggs so all of them would eat together (Dad's shepherd friend, the little girl and Dad). After Dad milked the sheep and his friend finished milking his sheep as they always did every evening, they sat down to eat.

When they finished dad told his friend it's time to give the little girl her medicine. When he went to give her the spoonful of medicine she starting crying. My dad stopped, with his hand trembling, and decided to taste this medicine. The medicine was very bitter, so he and his friend decided they would give it to her once every three days instead of everyday because dad told his friend, "This medicine is so bitter that it will destroy her stomach." After about a week dad asked his friend to go ask the village doctor (not the original doctor) what he thought about giving the medicine every third day instead of every day. The doctor told his friend, "Congratulations," you made a wise decision! If you had given her medicine every day she would have already died and you two young men would have been very upset.

Continue to give the medicine to her every third day and with the good feeding she is getting from the farm she will get stronger and stronger. Dad and his friend were relieved that they made the correct decision and continued to give her the medicine every third day but made sure that she had plenty of food every day.

After she finished all the medication it was only 20 days before dad would be moving his flock to higher grounds. This was the routine for dad and several other shepherds in that area. From late autumn to May they would take their flock to lower grounds away from the cold and snow of the mountains. In May they would again move their flock back to higher grounds to protect them from the heat and for available grass to feed on. Dad explained to the little girl that he would be leaving in about 20 days and would return in late autumn. He asked her if she wanted to go home now and she said, "No, I want to stay until you leave, and when you come back next year I want to come back and help you." The little girl returned to complete health in just under 3 months through proper nutrition and was able to live a happy and healthy life.

The final story I will share is a reminder that we don't have to be rich to help someone; there is always someone that is worse off than us. Two years after we arrived in America we opened a restaurant. My parents managed to run this restaurant knowing almost no English, and working from the time it opened at 11 a.m. until closing time, which was 2 a.m. They did all of the preparation, cooking, taking orders from customers, washing dishes and even mopping the floors at the end of each day. We didn't have much. We lived in a trailer without air-conditioning and without a television set. As I told my two children several times, the American dream is possible, but it takes a lot of hard work. This is especially true for immigrants like us because we started with nothing, as I imagine many immigrants do.

Both of my parents were philanthropist. I remember my mom used to give some customers extra food on their plate if she thought they didn't have enough money, or hold the baby so the young couple could enjoy their dinner. The most profound example that I remember was not one instance; it happened repeatedly over many days. It involved my dad helping an older man on a bicycle. The man would ride his bicycle to our parking lot, go to the trash bin outside, and immerse himself partially in it to find food. He would pick out pizza slices, bites of hamburgers, etc.

My dad would always run outside when he saw him and use the very little English he knew to convince the man to get out of the dumpster and come in and set at our table! We had a round table that our family and friends would set at in the very front of the restaurant. He would order the guy food and drink and set with him while he ate. Being a typical teenager, I was horrified that Dad would bring this man in and set him at our table. He smelled like urine, and he was very dirty; I was embarrassed. Looking back, I am ashamed that I felt that way. My dad, like all of us, was not a perfect man, but he always had compassion for the needy. My parents were also always thankful for the opportunity to come to America and better their lives.

With these true stories in mind, be a blessing to someone working hard to make it but having difficulty because his or her job isn't that great yet. Be mindful of people in minimum wage jobs that are working very hard to provide for themselves and their families. Here are some ideas on how to bless the hard working people that probably need some extra help:

- If your church is having a Christmas dinner, buy extra tickets and give them to someone you know is a hard working person but could use a night out but cannot afford it.

- Prepare a basket of the type of food you and your family would buy at the grocery store and give to someone you know is struggling.
- Purchase gift certificates at the same restaurant you prefer to eat at and give to a family that may not be able to afford that restaurant.
- Ask a server or a cook that you speak to often when you go out to eat what size shoes they wear. You would be surprised how many people would love a great pair of shoes to work in so their feet don't hurt, but end up getting the cheap shoes so they will have enough money for groceries or rent.
- Give a meaningful tip to the server at an inexpensive restaurant. Why should you give three times the tip to the server at an expensive restaurant for bringing you a more expensive meal? My son actually encouraged me to consider tipping in this manner. It's a blessing to have your grown children start challenging you to think more mindfully of others.

Hospitality is another good, healthy practice. Hospitality is actually giving also. I often exchange invitations with my friends from Cyprus and Greece to have coffee together. We will always say we are having coffee together, but we don't necessarily have coffee; we often have other drinks like tea or hot chocolate. When Greeks have you over for "coffee," there will be something served with it. It could be nuts, fresh fruit, or some type of sweet, but you will be offered something to eat. To do otherwise would show you to be a bad host! Also, you don't ask your guest if they want something; you just bring it to them.

In Greece, most of the time you are invited to come for coffee, but it's okay if you drop by without an invitation. When you arrive you will be asked to come in and set down; standing is not an option, and there will be a time commitment here. The host makes their guest feel at home and would never even slightly hint that they were being inconvenienced unless it was a dire emergency. If there are other family members at home, the customary etiquette is for those family members to rise and welcome the person to their home, and this includes children. Children are taught to properly greet the guests, show respect, and excuse themselves if they choose to leave the room.

The host asks, "What would you like to drink? Or how do you like your coffee?" The host never asks, "Do you want something to drink?" The host will name the options and then go to the kitchen to prepare the drinks. As I said earlier, some type of food to compliment the coffee (or other drink) will be brought out. The first time my husband went with me to Greece, we took him to meet my relatives; I could tell he was out of his comfort zone. Every relative we went to visit would, as he calls it, "Make me eat more food," which he was not use to.

Most of the time he was glad to eat what they offered because he loves Greek food, but there were a couple of times that he did not care for the selection. One of those memorable moments for my husband, that he will tell over and over again, was when we visited my aunt Olga. She had made dessert with figs, and she gave us a fig each, along with our coffee and water. My husband had never eaten a fig, much less a fig baked and drenched in sugary-honey syrup. It was a struggle for him to down it! Most of the time the food is placed in front of you to choose what you like but during this visit, my aunt wanted my husband to try her delicious dessert she made herself. Being the awesome person my American husband truly is, he did not want to hurt her feelings and managed to down it without demonstrating what he really thought about it.

Recently, my son and his lovely wife went to Greece, and this was my daughter-in-law's first visit to Greece. Because my son remembered the times he spent in my village Lafka, he wanted to take his wife and show her how beautiful it truly is. Lafka is an old, small village community nestled up against majestic mountains at the far-end of the valley containing Stymfalia Lake. We stopped in to say hello to my first cousin Demetra. We did not call her first, but just dropped by unannounced. She invited us up to her veranda insisting we sit down, and she went in the kitchen. A few minutes later she brought out her homemade Easter cookies, (it was right after Easter) glasses of cold water, and she asked how we all like our coffee. She went back in the kitchen and finished the coffee and brought it out on a serving tray (the proper way to serve in Greece). My daughter-in-law was blown away with Demetra's hospitality. After we left and got in the car to go back to Korinthos, she said, I cannot believe your cousin did all that and she doesn't know me, that was very nice, and I really needed that coffee and the Easter cookies were great."

How does this relate to health you ask? Part of the entire health endeavor is cultivating friends. Friends should enrich our lives and improve our health. If you are in a toxic kind of friendship, one that makes you feel bad about yourself, it's best to get away from that relationship. We all have our bad days, but we should not have constant negativity and complaints. God wants us to live happy and productive lives, and health is a major component of that kind of life.

The kind of hospitality I'm describing is not unique to Greece. If we take a look at the Holy Bible, the Word of God, we will see that type of hospitality from the Old Testament to the New Testament. Let's take a look at a couple of scripture verses:

"Come in, O blessed of the Lord! Why do you stand outside? For I have prepared the house, and a place for the camels." Genesis 24:31 (NKJV)

"Do not forget to entertain strangers, for by so doing some have unwittingly entertained angels." Hebrews 13:2 (NKJV)

Make connection between taking time to show hospitality and the time to prepare good food versus drive through windows!

CHAPTER TWENTY-TWO

Learning from Other Cultures

Traveling abroad is both a privilege and responsibility. How we behave and how we interact with the citizens of the host county presents them with a representation of what American culture and values look like. If you are disrespectful and hard for them to deal with, you demonstrate to the world that our country (you, me, your friends and family) and culture is disrespectful. You are representing both your country and countrymen, so represent us well. We have heard it over and over again, "It's not what we say, but how we act that people remember." I think it's both what we say and how we act, because they are listening and watching to learn our culture.

My husband took me to France in 2013 for our 35th anniversary. I had always heard stories about the French people being rude and not liking Americans, so I prepared myself to be confronted with unpleasant and rude people. To my surprise, the people of France are very nice to Americans, and very helpful. Thank God because I fell in love with France and it's people. Paris took my breath away!!! I loved all of those buildings with their architectural details. All those huge, beautiful cathedrals that were over 800 years old! They know how to preserve their historic buildings. I did have a not so pleasant experience at the Palace of Versailles from a group of people from a certain non-indigenous culture (I will not mention the nationality because

I do not want my readers to possibly get the wrong impression from this article). This group of people was pushing me in every room we visited. It was very crowded that day, and I guess they were in a hurry. I actually had to remove a ladies fist off the middle of my back at one point, and I also turned around to tell her to stop. Ever since that day when I see a person from that culture, I associate them with that group. It's unfair to do that because one group of people in a palace should not influence my opinion for an entire culture.

My husband does an excellent job showing the world that Americans are respectful people, because he understands it is important to respect others, and he shows it abroad. The Greeks absolutely love him! He greets everyone in the Greek language (even if the person knows English), he has a smile on his face, and when we are at a restaurant or a coffee shop he speaks his Greek. Many Greeks have difficulty understanding him the first time he speaks, but he repeats it, and you would not believe the smile on their faces. Don't have the attitude that another culture should act, look, eat, or dress like your culture. If that were the case the world would be boring and you would be better off staying at home looking at yourself in the mirror. You are visiting another country for the cultural experience, not to find another land with the same culture as yours.

My son loves traveling abroad, and has always stressed the importance of representing America well. He also gives his mother advice. It's a blessing to have your child give you advice. Most people in Greece and other countries will not have the opportunity to visit America. Most people in other countries form their opinion from what is said in the media or from an interaction with a visiting foreigner, so display your best behavior and represent your country well. So you ask, "What does this article have to do with health?" Other cuisines, like the Mediterranean/

Greek cuisine, are healthier than our western cuisine. We should be more open to try their food and learn how they prepare it so we can use some of their healthy methods in our kitchen. I encourage you to go abroad, and enjoy the experience—the people, the culture, the food!

But first learn some basic communication in their language like "Hello, how are you" and, "Thank you." Don't be arrogant and demand that others try to speak English to you; it's their country for crying out loud! Do you expect to have to speak German, Italian, or Russian in your own city? Probably not! If you don't make any attempt to at least start conversations and basic greetings in the native language, you will miss out on the opportunity to learn and be a part of a new culture. The best way to learn something is by interaction. Learning a new language (even a few words) and interacting with a different culture is exercise for the brain. Remember, the person speaking to you in English is using their second or third language, so don't use slang and speak English slow and clear. Make a little effort, and you will have a lot of wonderful memories to share with your family and friends.

You can live like a "Laukioti" (a person that lives in Lafka) without living in Lafka! The Lafka way of life is incredibly simple once you start taking out the trash. After you have taken the trash out:

- Eat legumes such as beans, lentils, and peas 4 times a week.
- Go semi-vegetarian. A semi-vegetarian includes meat occasionally.
- Eat lots of fruit that are in season.
- Make the vegetables the main course, and the meat a side.
- Use only extra virgin olive oil.

- Eat wild caught fish 2 times a week.
- Eat fermented foods such as Greek yogurt often. Yogurt should not have added sugar, please read the ingredients, and it must say "live culture bacteria" on the label.
- Make lunch the biggest meal of the day.
- Eat raw nuts daily, especially walnuts and almonds.
- Drink a small glass of red wine with your evening meal unless contraindicated by your faith, health, or family history.
- Do some form of exercise daily.
- Drink plenty of purified water.
- Hang out with positive people
- Feed your spirit

CHAPTER TWENTY-THREE

Nutrition Analysis

Please write down everything you eat and drink for the next three days as accurately as possible. Also include coffee, alcoholic beverages, soda, candy bars, etc. Explain in detail how the food was prepared, e.g. instead of writing chicken breast.

Comments: Writing down what you eat can help you identify your good and your bad habits.

Day 1

Breakfast:

Lunch:

Dinner:

Snacks:

Day 2

Breakfast:

Lunch:

Dinner:

Snacks:

Day 3

Breakfast:

Lunch:

Dinner:

Snacks:

Is the above an accurate representation of your overall diet? If no, please do the analysis on a week that represents your normal diet.

Comments: A daily food journal will help you see what you really eat. A good journal will show specific habits that may not be healthy, for example: You may realize that when you watch television you eat more or may find that you have become a garbage disposal by eating what the kids left on the table or that little bit in the pan that is not worth saving.

What time do you eat your last meal?

Comments: anywhere from 1-3 hours before bedtime is a good rule of thumb. You should experiment different times to figure out what works for you. Here's some of the possible reasons you should not eat a big meal before going to bed: indigestion, reflux, and Chronic Obstructive Pulmonary Disease (COPD). You can add a bedtime snack to your routine as long as it's a healthy snack.

Do you cook at home most of the time?

Comments: you can dine out occasionally and stay healthy (see the chapter, Dine Out Without Pigging Out). There is a connection between food and disease. To optimize your nutrition and reduce the chances of getting disease or reduce the time to recovery you must cook at home the majority of the time. Greek cooking consists mainly of fresh ingredients. The dishes changed with seasonal bounty in my village of Lafka. Whatever was in season was what we ate. It was packed with nutrition because it was fresh; we never ate processed food. The solution to our health crisis in America is to go back and eat like the Greeks did 40-50 years ago.

What oil to you use to cook with?
Comments: Use extra virgin olive oil as your primary cooking oil. Here's some of the benefits of extra virgin olive oil: Helps with longevity, makes you feel full thus may help with weigh loss, helps reduce inflammation, may help with anti-aging, and more.

How many glasses of purified water do you drink per day?
Comments: Drink 6-8 glasses of purified water per day, depending on your size and weight. Water flushes out toxins, carries nutrients to your cells, allows your kidneys to function properly, and allows easier elimination.

How many servings of fresh or frozen fruits do you eat per day?
Comments: Eat at least 3 servings of fruits per day but remember more is better. Tip on how can you increase your daily intake: always have fruit washed and ready to grab and eat. Try a different fruit once a week because as we know variety is a benefit to overall health. No single fruit provides all of the nutrients you need.

How many servings of fresh or frozen vegetables do you eat per day?
Comments: Eat at least 3 servings of vegetables per day but remember more is better. Tip on how you can increase your daily intake: Make more vegetable soups, salads, stir fry and roasted vegetables and decrease the amount of pasta and breads in your diet.

How many days do you eat legumes?

Comments: Legumes provide a variety of nutrients such as protein, excellent source of complex carbohydrates, folate, thiamine and magnesium. What are legumes? beans, peas, and lentils. It has been said that studies have shown that people who eat more legumes have lower risk of heart disease. We ate legumes 3 times a week or more at my village when I was living in Greece. It must be one of the reasons my dad at 98 was told by his doctor that he has a heart of a 40 year old.

How many servings of complex carbohydrates (bran, steel cut oats, quinoa, peas, lentils, potatoes, kidney beans, chick peas, pinto beans, broccoli, spinach, green beans, apples, pears, cucumbers, yams, asparagus, prunes, beans, carrots, buckwheat, wheat etc.) do you eat per day?

Comments: Carbohydrates fuel physical activity and are an important part of a healthy diet. Simple carbohydrates, such as table sugar, should be avoided. Simple carbohydrates cause quicker spikes in blood sugar (sugar rush) that leaves you with no energy quickly. Complex carbohydrates sustain energy over longer periods. Vegetables, whole grain products and fruits are good sources of complex carbohydrates.

Do you drink sodas or diet sodas?

Comments: Sugar is bad for your health! Eliminate all sugary drinks, including those with sugar substitutes. There are 40 different names of sugar, and I have them listed under my "Healthy Solutions to a Healthy Weight." Sugar substitutes are bad also. You are best to eliminate sodas from your diet.

How many refined sugar items (candy bars, donuts, cakes, etc.) do you eat per day?

Comments: We all know by now that refined sugar items are bad for your health. As I mention in "Your health is your wealth," investing in your health is a wise decision, and one that leads to optimal health for a long time. You are what you eat in terms of health. Do you want to be in a better mood, increase energy, reduce weight if you need to, reduce the chances of getting disease, etc.? It's your choice.

How many fast food items or processed meats (hamburgers, hot dogs, salami, bologna, frozen dinners, canned foods etc.) do you eat per day?
Comments: It's not rocket science to understand that fast foods can cause you health issues. Let's be honest, do we really think that these items have high quality ingredients, and what about chemical additives? You and your family deserve the best nutrition to build and maintain health.

Do you smoke or use tobacco products?
Comments: Smoking damages health! We all know that but how can someone stop? Here's a suggestion may help you stop smoking; go to a health food store and ask for an herb that other people have used to kick the habit, but consult with your doctor first if you are on any medication. Also, read all the possible side effects of that herb.

How many days per week do you exercise for a minimum of 30 minutes?
Comments: Exercise is a very important component to wellness. I recommend 3-4 days a week for 30 minutes to one hour per day. Being consistent is more important than amount of time per day. It's important to start slow and build up your strength to avoid injury. Rather than saying how can you add exercise to a busy schedule, identify activities that you value less than your health and eliminate those time-wasters. Replace them with physical activities that support good health and actually energize you to engage in life even more. . Exercise does not necessarily need to

be done in a gym. Some other ways to get physical activity are: a brisk walk, biking, swimming, jogging, and gardening. Last but not least, if you are under a doctor's care please consult your physician first before starting an exercise program.

Stress may be affecting your health, what is your inner dialogue? Are you into a positive or negative dialogue? How much time per day do you devote to prayer and God's Word?
Comments: Spiritual well- being is also important to wellness. Consider reading out of your bible daily, and praying daily. Prayer does not have to be done only in the closet; it can be done in your car, outside, at your morning break at work, etc. I can tell you from personal experience my life is less stressful because I have learned through God's Word and through prayer (talking to God) to not stress over the little things and to give God the things that I cannot handle. If your inner dialogue is negative I suggest you find positive quotes; print them, and post them on your bathroom mirror. This method worked for me when I had an enormous stressful period and nobody could help me other than God. I praise God for teaching me to rely on Him, to have faith in Him that He will handle the things I cannot, and to give me wisdom to know the difference.

CHAPTER TWENTY-FOUR

Recipes for Health

Navy beans (fasolada in Greek)

16 oz. dry navy beans: soaked in water in the refrigerator for 10-24 hours
1 large minced onion sautéed in ½ cup extra virgin olive oil.
1 fresh tomato, chopped
½ cup tomato sauce
3 1/2 cup water
2 -3 bay leaves
Salt and pepper

In slow-cooker on low for 6 hours

Navy bean salad (fasolada salata):

16 oz. dry navy beans: soaked in water in the refrigerator for 10-24 hours
1 Cup of extra virgin olive oil
3 ½ Cups water
2-3 Bay leaves
Cook in slow cooker on low for 6 hours.

In individual serving bowls or a big bowl add beans along with:
Chopped tomatoes
Chopped cucumbers

Chopped green onion or red onion
Chopped fresh spinach or chopped parsley
Chopped green peppers or chopped banana peppers
Drizzle a little extra virgin olive oil on the top
Fresh squeezed lemon juice to taste
Season with salt & Pepper
Combine all ingredients and serve with fresh whole wheat bread,
Kalamata olives, and feta cheese. If you prefer a cold salad, cover,
and refrigerate for about 2 hours before serving.

Enjoy!

Lima Beans recipe:

12 oz. package of frozen lima beans
1/3-cup extra virgin olive oil
1 small onion chopped
1/3-cup tomato sauce
1 and 1/3cup water
Oregano
Chopped parsley

In a medium sized pot sauté onions in olive oil. Add all other
ingredients to the pot and bring to a boil. Reduce heat to low, and
cover beans, let simmer for 15-25 minutes, stirring occasionally.
Options: add Romano or Parmesan cheese before serving.

Serve along with:
Stir fry with rice or pasta
Baked potatoes
Baked sweet potatoes
Salads
Fried potatoes
Rice
Pasta salad

Kidney beans in the crock-pot:

16 oz. dry kidney beans soaked in water for 12-24 hours and rinsed.

¾ Cup extra virgin olive oil
1 small or medium onion grated
2-3 cloves of garlic chopped

Chop celery, including the leafy part on the top.
2-3 Fresh carrots pilled and chopped in small round pieces
Parsley
Juice of 3 fresh lemons
Sea salt & Pepper
4 Cups of water

Sauté the onion and garlic in the olive oil. Add all the ingredients in the crock-pot and cook on low temperature for 6-8 hours.

Serving options: Add small cooked pasta or cooked orzo or cooked rice when the beans are finished cooking. Tip: the kidney beans can be frozen and thawed at a later date to add to your chili dinner.

Pinto Beans:

16 oz. of dry pinto beans soaked in water in refrigerator overnight

1 chopped onion sautéed in ½ cup of extra virgin olive oil
1 fresh tomato chopped
½ cup tomato sauce
3 - cups of water
2 bay leaves
Parsley
Cilantro
Oregano

Mix all the ingredients together and pour into the crock -pot.

Cook on low for 6 hours.

Lentil soup

1-cup lentils
Cover with water and cook for 1 minute
Rinse the lentils
In a pot add the lentils
1 cup chopped onion
2 chopped carrots
1 tsp. chopped garlic
1 chopped potato
½ cup tomato sauce
½ tsp. paprika
2 TBL red wine vinegar
½ cup olive oil
2 bay leaves
4 cups water
Oregano
Bring to boil, reduce to low and cook for approximately 30 minutes.

Chicken and Vegetable soup:

2/3 Cup extra virgin olive oil
1 Chopped onion
2-3 cloves of garlic chopped
1-2 fresh zucchini chopped

1 ½ to 2 cups cooked roasted chicken and cut in small pieces
1 Cup tomato sauce
1 fresh tomato chopped or 1 cup of chopped cherry tomatoes

Frozen peas or frozen Lima beans, 10 oz
2-3 Fresh carrots chopped
Oregano
1 Cup chopped Italian parsley
1 Teaspoon paprika
½ Teaspoon Cinnamon
Red pepper flakes to your taste
Sea salt
Black pepper

In a large pot, sauté the onions, garlic, and zucchini in the olive oil until the onions are tender. Add all the other ingredients and enough water to cover the vegetables. Bring to a boil, then reduce the heat to low, cover and simmer for 30 minutes or until the vegetables are done.

Season to taste with sea salt and freshly ground black pepper

*Other vegetable options are: chopped potato, and chopped sweet potato.

Serving option: sprinkle your favorite cheese on the top before serving.

Egg rolls made easy:

Cooked chicken cut in small pieces
Carrots shredded
Cabbage shredded
Organic soy sauce
Mix all of the above well.

Egg roll wrappers

Sweet and sour sauce

Lay the wrapper with the one angle facing you on a clean flat surface. Brush the four corners with water. Spoon a heaping tablespoon of filling near the bottom corner. Lift the corner up and start rolling it to half way up. Fold over the right and left sides to the center. Continue to roll it all the way to the other corner. Seal the corner by brushing it with water.

Oil to fry the egg rolls: I use olive oil on medium heat but it splatters so be careful if you use it. In a skillet set on medium heat, fry the eggs rolls on all sides until golden brown using tongs to turn them. Serve with sweet and sour sauce.

Oven-Baked Salmon

One whole wild caught salmon
(Ingredients: wild caught salmon)
Juice of two fresh limes or lemons
Dried oregano
½ Cup extra virgin olive oil
1 Teaspoon paprika
Fresh coriander or fresh mint or fresh parsley
4-5 cloves of garlic chopped
Salt & Pepper

Directions
Preheat oven to 450 degrees F.

Place salmon, with the skin side down, on a baking dish lined with parchment paper. Season the salmon with salt, pepper and paprika. Add on the top of the salmon evenly, chopped garlic, oregano, extra virgin olive oil, and fresh herb of your choice.

Bake uncovered for approximately 20 minutes (check it in 15 minutes). Place on broil for a few minutes at the end for a golden brown color but check it constantly to prevent it from burning.

Meatballs:

1 lb. organic ground beef or ground bison
Dry Mint and dry oregano
Fresh oregano chopped (optional)
3 slices of Ezekiel breadcrumbs
1 egg
1 tsp. vinegar
Sea salt & ground pepper
1 Small onion grated
1 tsp. Dijon mustard
1/3 cup Parmesan or Romano cheese

Note: if they seem a little dry add ¼ cup extra virgin olive oil

Mix all except ground beef. Add beef and mix. Refrigerate for 1 hour

Form into balls (about ¼ cup full each) and coat each one with extra virgin olive oil. Bake on 350F for approximately 30 minutes or until no longer pink in the middle.

Optional:

When meatballs are done add salsa and Parmesan cheese, cook for 5 minutes or until salsa is warm.

Baked chicken:

Whole chicken free of antibiotics and growth hormones
¼ Cup Dijon mustard
½ Cup extra virgin olive oil
1 Tablespoon dried oregano
1-Teaspoon Turmeric
1-Teaspoon cinnamon

½ Cup water
Juice of two fresh lemons
Honey

Heat oven to 350o

Place the chicken whole in a baking pan with ½ cup of water. Cook for one hour, remove from pan and discard the drippings. Mix all other ingredients except the water (I use a bullet). Pour the mixture over the chicken with breast up, and add the water at the bottom of the pan. Cover the chicken with parchment paper first and than aluminum foil and bake on 375o for one hour. Take chicken of the oven. Cut chicken in half, and turn it with cavity of chicken down. Cut slices in the breast, spoon juices from the bottom of the pan on the top of the chicken, drizzle a little honey and put it back in the oven on 400o uncovered until golden brown. Bon appetite

Summer chili

Ingredients:
1 lb. organic ground beef
½ Cup tomato sauce
1 16 oz. organic mild or medium salsa
(You can add 1 fresh tomato when they are in season also)
1 cup kidney beans, drained
1 Medium onion grated
3 stalks of diced celery
1 Green pepper, diced
(You can add yellow and/or red peppers if you have them also).
1 Diced zucchini
½ teaspoon chili powder (use more if you prefer it hotter)
½ teaspoon turmeric
Dried oregano

½ teaspoon organic sugar
½ cup red wine
1-½ cups purified water
Salt & Pepper to taste

Brown the ground beef. Add all the remaining ingredients, bring to a boil, reduce to simmer and cook for approximately 30 minutes. If the chili becomes overly dry, add a little more water.

Serving suggestions: sprinkle Parmesan cheese or organic cheddar cheese. Homemade bread, or Kettle chips are great as a side.

Roasted Vegetables:

4 Potatoes cut in chunks
1 Green pepper sliced
1 Red onion sliced in thick rings
2 Zucchini sliced thick
5 Carrots cut 1' thick
Juice of 1 fresh orange
Juice of 3 fresh lemons
1 Cup extra virgin olive oil
Oregano
Parsley
Sea salt and Pepper

Bake on 400o for approximately 45 minutes (stir the vegetables often during the cooking process).

Sweet Potato fries:

Turn oven on 450o
Slice the sweet potatoes thin or cut them to look like fries
Line cookie sheet with parchment paper

In a bowl toss sweet potatoes with just enough extra virgin olive oil to coat. Sprinkle with a little paprika. Bake until golden brown; turning them once the topside is done to brown the other side, approximately 20 minutes.

Stir fry with a Greek twist:

Red onion, chopped
Carrots, chopped
Yellow squash, chopped
Zucchini, chopped
Red Peppers, sliced
Green Peppers, sliced
Broccoli, chopped
(You may add other vegetables also)
Extra virgin olive oil
Organic soy sauce

If you want to add meat add cooked, left over roast or chicken chopped.

Drizzle extra virgin olive oil to coat the bottom of the pan, add the vegetables and stir often for about 2-3 minutes
Add the organic soy sauce and continue to stir for a few more minutes until the vegetables are done and the meat is hot.
Taste the vegetables and see if you want to add more soy sauce
Do not add salt because soy sauce has sodium in it already.

Serving suggestions:
Add it on the top of cooked rice.
Add it on the top of cooked spaghetti or pasta and sprinkle with Parmesan cheese.

Roasted Greek Potatoes:

Preheat over to 400o

6-7 medium potatoes, peeled and cut in quarters
1-Teaspoon Dijon mustard
Thyme (optional)
2 Teaspoons dry oregano
Juice of 1- 1/2 fresh lemon
½ Cup extra virgin olive oil
1-Cup water
Salt and pepper

In a bowl, whisk together all ingredients with the exception of the potatoes. In a large bowl add the potatoes and the other ingredients. Coat the potatoes well, and cook them for approximately 1 hour and 10 minutes or until golden brown. Be sure to stir the potatoes every 15-20 minutes.

Fruity spinach salad with the option to add left over chicken or turkey:

8 oz. fresh organic spinach washed (approximately 4 servings)
2 cup chopped organic apples
1-2 sliced fresh oranges
1 cup frozen, thawed blue berries
½ cup pomegranate if in season, optional
½ cup dried cranberries
1 cup diced block cheese
2-3 chopped fresh organic carrots
½ cup chopped walnuts

Dressing:
¼ cup fresh lemon juice

½ cup extra virgin olive oil
Oregano
1 Teaspoon sea salt
Ground black pepper
Mix in a bullet or with an electric mixer

Homemade Bread:

*2 Cups organic flour sifted
2 Cups whole-wheat non-GMO flour sifted
1 Teaspoon sea salt
1 Teaspoon dried yeast
2 Tablespoons of honey
¼ Cup extra virgin olive oil
Warm water as needed

Using a large bowl, add the flour, sea salt and dry yeast and mix well. Make a well in the middle and add the honey, oil, and some warm water. Start to knead the mixture and add water as needed for the dough to form but still be a little sticky. Knead the dough for about 2-3 minutes. The dough should be a little sticky but not too sticky that you can't handle it. Place the dough in a bowl 2-3 times larger than the dough that has been greased with olive oil, and turn it once to grease the top. Cover and let rise in a warm place until doubled, about 1-1/2 hours. Grease with olive oil and lightly flour the baking dish or use parchment paper that has been greased with olive oil. Place the dough in the pan and spread evenly. Make 3-4 slits on the top with a knife. Cover and let rise until doubled, about 30-45 minutes.

Bake on 350o for 45 minutes to 1 hour or until golden brown. When it's cooled down wrap it with parchment paper and place it in a plastic bag. Keep the leftover bread in the refrigerator.

Note: Using the same recipe I also make individual buns instead of one loaf to use for our egg sandwiches or as hamburger buns. The buns can be frozen wrapped in parchment paper and in zip lock bags for later use.

*You can use all whole-wheat flour, but if you and your family are not use to the texture yet it's best to mix it with regular flour for a few weeks.

ABOUT THE AUTHOR

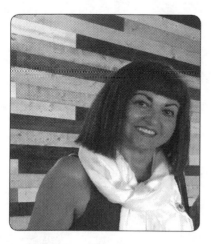

Rena Ayyelina is a certified nutritional consultant in natural medicine. Mrs. Ayyelina and her family immigrated to the United States when she was eleven years old. Her first introduction to nutrition and its relationship to health and well-being was through her village of Lafka, Korinthias. While living in America, Mrs. Ayyelina ate the typical American diet for 13 years due to living in a restaurant environment. As an adult, she started making radical changes in her diet while carrying her first child to ensure proper nutrition for her baby. She continued to make improvements to her cooking methods and food selections to improve her family's nutrition and also began educating friends and relatives that were willing to hear the relationship between nutrition and well-being. Convinced that nutrition is, in many cases, the answer to America's health crisis, Mrs. Ayyelina created a health and wellness Facebook page to reach as many people as possible with her passion for promoting health through nutrition. This book shares her journey and passion toward improved health and vitality in a genuine, down-to-earth, common sense reflection on her Mediterranean village lifestyle.

Printed in the United States
By Bookmasters